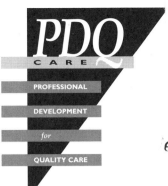

 STANDARD LOA**

Please return or rene·

Promoting the
Health of the Nation

Reader material selected and compiled by

Sally Kendall BSc (Hons) PhD RHV RGN
Professor of Primary Health Care Nursing, Faculty of Health Studies, Buckinghamshire College of
Brunel University, Buckinghamshire

Sandra Lask BA (Hons) MScHealthEd RGN RNT PGCE
Lecturer, RCN Institute, Royal College of Nursing, London

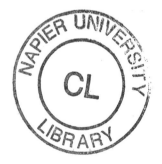
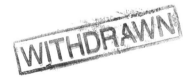
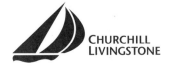
CHURCHILL
LIVINGSTONE

NEW YORK EDINBURGH LONDON MADRID MELBOURNE SAN FRANCISCO TOKYO 1997

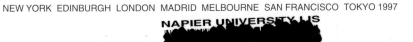

CHURCHILL LIVINGSTONE
Medical Division of Pearson Professional Limited

Distributed in the United States of America by
Churchill Livingstone, 650 Avenue of the Americas,
New York, N.Y. 10011, and by associated companies,
branches and representatives throughout the world.

First published 1997

ISBN 0 443 05225 5

British Library Cataloguing in Publication Data
A catalogue record for this book is available from the British Library.

Library of Congress Cataloguing in Publication Data
A catalogue record for this book is available from the
Library of Congress.

Note
Medical knowledge is constantly changing. As new information
becomes available, changes in treatment, procedures, equipment
and the use of drugs become necessary. The editors/authors/
contributors and the publishers have, as far as it is possible,
taken care to ensure that the information given in this text
is accurate and up to date. However, readers are strongly
advised to confirm that the information, especially with regard
to drug usage, complies with latest legislation and standards of
practice.

Printed by Bell and Bain Ltd., Glasgow

For Churchill Livingstone:

Editorial director: Mary Law
Project manager: Valerie Burgess
Project development editor: Valerie Bain
Design direction: Judith Wright
Project controller: Pat Miller
Pre-press desktop operator: Gerard Heyburn
Sales promotion executive: Hilary Brown

Contents

Acknowledgements

Grateful acknowledgement is made to the following sources for permission to reproduce the offprints contained in the Reader:

The Royal Society of Health for: Mitchell J 1982 Looking after ourselves: an individual responsibility? Royal Society of Health Journal 102(4): 169–173 (Offprint 1). Tones BK 1981 Health education: prevention or subversion? Royal Society of Health Journal 101(3): 114–117 (Offprint 2).

The Health Visitors' Association for: Harrison J 1994 Every picture tells the story. Health Visitor 67(2): 66–67 (Offprint 3). Jackson C 1992 Community mothers: trick or treat? Health Visitor 65(6): 199–201 (Offprint 4).

Her Majesty's Stationery Office for: extracts from *Targeting Practice: the Contribution of Nurses, Midwives and Health Visitors* (The Health of the Nation) 1993, pp. 28–30, 56–57 (Offprint 5) and *Purchasing for the Health of the Nation* leaflet (Offprint 16). Crown copyright is reproduced with the permission of the Controller of Her Majesty's Stationery Office.

The Guardian for Ham C 1994 And today's remedy will be … Guardian 6 August (Offprint 6) and Mullin J, Myers P 1994 Woman accused of Abbie abduction 'could not cope after shame of losing own baby' Guardian 20 July (Offprint 10). Copyright Guardian.

The BMJ Publishing Group for: Imperial Cancer Research Fund OXCHECK Study Group 1995 Effectiveness of health checks conducted by nurses in primary care: final results of the OXCHECK study. British Medical Journal 310: 1009–1104 (Offprint 7). Family Heart Study Group (Wood et al) 1994 Randomised controlled trial evaluating cardiovascular screening and intervention in general practice: principal results of British family heart study. British Medical Journal 308: 313–320 (Offprint 8).

Oxford University Press for: Schofield M et al 1993 Skin cancer: do early childcare centres provide protection? Health Promotion International 8(4): 243–247 (Offprint 9).

Carfax Publishing Company for: Hoggett P 1993 What is community mental health. Journal of Interprofessional Care 7(3): 201–209 (Offprint 11). Carfax Publishing Company, PO Box 25, Abingdon, Oxfordshire OX14 3UE.

The Child Accident Prevention Trust for: The picture of childhood accidents: questionnaire (Offprint 12) in *Preventing Accidents to Children: a Training Resource for Health Visitors* 1991: 26–27.
Note: The picture of childhood accidents: information sheet (Offprint 13) in *Preventing Accidents to Children: a Training Resource for Health Visitors* 1991: 28–31 is based on information supplied by sources as listed in offprint.

Macmillan Press Limited for: Kendrick D 1994 Children's safety in the home: parents' possession and perceptions of the importance of safety equipment (Offprint 14). Public Health 108: 21–25.

The BMJ Publishing Group for: Roberts H 1991 Accident Prevention: a community approach. Health Visitor 64(7): 219–220 (Offprint 15).

R.S.H. 4 1982

Looking after ourselves: an individual responsibility?

JEANNETTE MITCHELL
Journalist, Times Health Supplement

IN THE last five years there has been increasing official enthusiasm for the notion that all of us could and should improve our own health by changing our life style. This paper argues that this initiative will not only fail to lead to any significant improvement in people's health, it is also profoundly anti-health. By encouraging people to see their problems as their own fault, attention is distracted from the social and economic roots of ill health and people's confidence to challenge the societal causes of illness undermined. Lay people are interested in their own health, but will not be encouraged to take greater control over it while medical practice maintains them in a position of passivity and ignorance. If health workers want to help people to take more control over their own health, they must challenge the self-help philosophy and examine their own practice to see how it could embody an alternative approach to prevention.

THE NEW PHILOSOPHY

THE CURRENT enthusiasm for 'life-stylism' has its origins in the mid 1970s around the time the International Monetary Fund intervened to tell the then Labour Government it had to cut back public expenditure. As the pressure to reduce state spending mounted, self-help was seen explicitly as a way of saving money. The first initiative towards establishing the legitimacy of the idea of self-help was taken not by the Department of Health, but by the House of Commons Expenditure Committee, which in November 1975, began an investigation into the money saving possibilities of preventive medicine. The primary conclusion of their report[1], published in 1977, was as follows:

"We have been convinced by our enquiry that substantial human and financial resources would be saved if greater emphasis were to be placed on prevention. This is not just a theoretical conclusion; it is literally a matter of life and death. Our recommendations cover organisation, training, advertising, finance, and *last but not least, self help*." (my italics)

The same ideas recur over and over again in official documents of the period. The Department of Health and Social Security's own booklet *Prevention and Health: Everybody's Business*[2], published some months before the Expenditure Committee's report, spelt out the new thinking:

"A great battle has been won, and at first sight victory seems complete, but a second look shows a different picture. More people can expect to live longer than in previous generations, but many still die prematurely or are for many years of their life dogged by avoidable ill health. . . . We all need to be more aware of how we can help ourselves, our families and the community as a whole to avoid illness and their consequences."

The booklet was essentially arguing that great leaps forward were made in the nineteenth century through improvements, in living standards, diet and sanitation. Today, although there have been enormous improvements in people's health there are a whole range of diseases which medicine cannot cure. A new initiative in prevention is required, except this time the problem is primarily not to do with environmental conditions, but people's individual life styles.

The official Government response to the Expenditure Committee report, a White Paper, *Prevention and Health*[3] published later in 1977, clearly rejected any notion that standards of health might be related to the material conditions under which people live and work:

"A rising standard of living, which has contributed to the improvement of the population's health in the past, cannot be expected to improve the position with regard to the modern scourges . . . In fact, unless habits can be changed, further increases in the standard of living may result in an increased prevalence of these diseases."

The White Paper even committed the Government to some increased spending on health education. Since then we have had the Health Education Council's *Look After Yourself* campaign and the Scottish Health Education Group's *Dying Scot*. The Department of Health has published glossy booklets on healthy eating and avoiding heart attacks. Words like 'life style' and 'health behaviour' are now on the lips of every ambitious health professional, and there is a growing research industry busily investigating why human beings (especially the ubiquitous social classes four and five) persist in the perverse pursuit of bad health.

PARTIAL TRUTHS

IF ALL this had simply been a money saving ploy, the new thinking might well have bitten the dust, especially as within the medical profession there must have been very ambiguous feelings about the criticism of high technology medicine implicit in it. But like many dangerous ideas, the new self-help ideology incorporates powerful, if partial truths, appealing to a growing spectrum of people critical of medicine as well as many health professionals.

Firstly, it appears that there is already considerable popular enthusiasm for what might loosely be described as 'self help'. There is a growing interest in physical fitness, self-care and mutual support groups. People are interested in knowing more about their own bodies and deciding for themselves how to meet their health care problems. The women's movement, for instance, has

LOOKING AFTER OURSELVES

been highly critical of the way in which doctors keep them in the dark about their own bodies and fail to consult them on crucial issues. Women's groups have learned to examine their own bodies and organised health courses with the aim of helping women do more for themselves and encounter doctors on more equal terms. But, although the women's movement has perhaps been the most vocal, similar criticisms of medicine have come from many other quarters. Pensioners, fed up with being told 'it's just your age' by doctors have also organised their own health courses. Ethnic minority groups who have found problems like sickle cell anaemia ignored or blamed on themselves have set up their own organisations to engage in health education and campaigning. In the trade union movement there has been a growing interest in health and safety issues. In some cases workers have conducted their own surveys on their health problems. Nowadays there are mutual suppport groups for people who face all kinds of common chronic health problems from tinnitus to psoriasis. Such groups are often engendered by a feeling that many doctors do not tell their patients much about their condition and indeed often have less useful advice about everyday ways of coping than fellow sufferers.

Secondly, those who argue for more prevention are absolutely right to emphasise that increasing investment in medical technology over the last twenty years has given rise to few dividends in terms of increases in life expectancy or cures for the modern killers, especially heart disease and cancer. Since the 1950s the graph of increasing life expectancy has flattened off. Survival rates in many forms of cancer are little better than they were twenty years ago, and doubts have also been cast on the efficacy of medical intervention in prolonging the lives of heart disease sufferers.

The emphasis on how much modern ill health is, by contrast, preventable must also be welcomed. We now know that 75 per cent of cancer is in principle avoidable and that a high proportion of heart disease could be prevented by changes in what we eat, by stopping smoking and reducing stress in our lives. The vast class differences in mortality and mobidity rates (see appendix) are themselves a testament to how much ill health is essentially preventable.

CLASS REALITY DENIED

SO IF the state is encouraging us to recognise the limitations of medicine in improving the general health of the population, pointing out how much ill health is preventable and suggesting that we all get involved in looking after ourselves for which there appears to be growing grass roots enthusiasm, why is the move to encourage self-help both incorrect and dangerous? The error lies in the assumption that health can be improved by the actions of individuals *on their own* and that because ill health is in principle preventable each of us as individual citizens can be held responsible for our own ill health. In rejecting this view there are three main points to be made:
(a) Many of the causes of illness, including the so-called life style diseases cancer and heart disease, though preventable by societal action are not the subject of individual choice. The mother whose child falls out of a tower block window, may well have been pressing the housing department for rehousing for years. The man who contracts mesothelioma may not have been told by his employer that the substance he was working with contained asbestos. The old lady who dies of hypothermia may well have been aware that her

supplementary benefit was not sufficient to keep her house properly warm, but have been unable to convince the social security office of this. What is in the air we breathe, our working conditions, our housing conditions, and the stress in our lives are often outside our individual control.
(b) Furthermore many areas of life which appear to be the subject of individual choice, in the jargon, matters of life style, like what we eat and how much we smoke are also the product of societal forces. We are all familiar with the argument about the tobacco industry. As the Black Report on *Inequalities in Health*[5], which argues that smoking cannot be taken as a fundamental cause of ill health but is a secondary symptom of deeper economic realities, points out:
"It is no good treating cigarette smoking as an aberrant or irresponsible behavioural response while society as a whole permits, even depends on, the widescale production and promotion of tobacco goods."
This argument is equally true of what we eat. Food is produced with profit not health in mind. 'Junk food' is most profitable precisely because it has got fewest good things in it and is designed to make you want to eat more of it. In a society which depends on the manufacture of health-destructive products from cars to tobacco, with a powerful advertising industry telling us we will be lesser people if we do not consume them, it is clearly contradictory for the Government to be telling us we should not be consuming these products.

Living standards are also a crucial influence on life style. For many pensioners and families on low incomes fresh fruit is these days a luxury. Working class families still consume far more bread and sugar than middle class families and white bread remains cheaper than wholemeal.
(c) It is nevertheless possible to argue that whatever the production process, it is a matter of individual choice whether you eat food that is bad for you, drink and smoke. How many times is it also said that because working class people spend money on unhealthy 'luxuries' like sweets, cakes, cigarettes and beer, the problem cannot be one of living standards. One reason is that people choose unhealthy luxuries because they cannot afford healthy ones like living in the suburbs, where the air is cleaner, or holidays abroad.

Questions of 'life style' are subject to even more subtle and profound influences than the activities of the advertising industry. How many sweets you give your kids may depend on how many hours you have to spend cooped up with them, which may in turn, be related to how many roads you have to cross to the nearest playground. There is no point in giving up smoking in order to live longer into a future without a job. It is very hard to do without sticky cakes if it is one of the few treats in your life. If you never have enough sleep because you work as an office cleaner and have to get up at six, you probably will not be inclined, nor have the time and energy to take up jogging.

Individual examples of the case against life-stylism may sound trivial, a cold pensioner here, an unemployed cigarette smoker there, until you bear in mind that they all add up to a pattern. It is on the whole the same people who work shifts, who are most likely to be unemployed, whose neighbourhood is likely to be heavily polluted, whose children tend to have accidents on the street, who have hazardous jobs, and for whom the future is grey.

Good health is possible when you have decent air to breathe, when you can afford to go on holiday, when

R.S.H. 4 1982   *JEANNETTE MITCHELL*

Occupational class and mortality in adult life
(men and married women by husband's occupation)
(15-64)

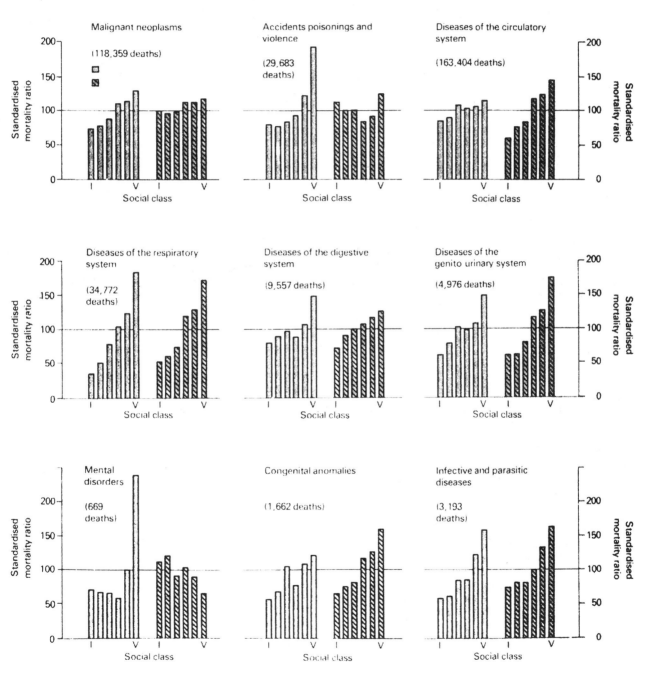

Source   Black Report into 'Inequalities in Health' DHSS 1980.
Occupational Mortality, 1970–72 HMSO 1978

you can choose what food to buy and have the time and energy to enjoy cooking it. When your children have somewhere safe to play, when you are warm, when you enjoy your work, when you have confidence in and look forward to the future. For most people in Britain today these are not possibilities. A million pensioners are so cold they are at risk of hypothermia. Three million people are unemployed. 6 million of Britain's 15 million children are being brought up at or on the margins of poverty. Ours is a class society in which the people with the least power suffer the worst health.

To most people the *dying Scot* and the *Look after yourself* cartoon man of the health education campaigns are an irrelevance. The recent Government booklet *Avoiding heart attacks*[6] encourages us to change our lives to give up smoking, eat better and reduce stress. It does not mention that twice as many men in unskilled jobs are likely to die of this 'executive' disease than in professional jobs, nor does it consider why people might be under stress.

When the White Paper *Prevention and Health* said "the problem of communicating effectively with people in social classes four and five is not a new one" it expressed a sentiment often heard from doctors and health educators exasperated by what appears to be the irrationality of those most at risk. But the message may well be falling on deaf ears because the message is nonsense. It may well be that those at the bottom of society appear to be such bad listeners because they have got enough on their plates without being told what to do by people who are out of touch with their life experience.

THE FECKLESS AT FAULT

ALTHOUGH Government publications and pronouncements deny the material origins of class inequalities in health, this does not mean they can be dismissed as irrelevant. Whatever the intention, the practical effect has been to encourage health care professionals and policy makers to see the preventable health problems of working class people as their own fault. Many doctors have always been inclined to blame the 'feckless' for their misfortunes. Whether it is inadequate child rearing practices, failure to attend family planning or ante-natal clinics, spending the week's wages on alcohol or giving the children too many sweets. Now, as the daily life style message is disseminated through the medical and popular press as well as in official publications, health professionals have every encouragement to intensify their inclination to victim blaming.

The effect is to make people feel guilty and to undermine any understanding of the social and economic causes of ill health by a systematic denial of people's class experience. Pensioners resent Government advice to keep warm when their problem is they cannot afford the heating bills. Already anxious mothers worried about making ends meet often come away from the doctor feeling even less confident when they are told they have not been looking after their children properly. Asian people to whom the Government had denied vitamin D in chapati flour, are made to feel guilty for not feeding their children a Western diet when their children get rickets.

A recent editorial in the Lancet[7] pointed out that self-help often means self-blame:

"As *Prevention and Health: Everybody's Business* implies, the other side of individual responsibility in health is blaming the individual if he or she gets sick. Given the persistent social inequalities in health, this seems a barely defensible position. Statements emphasising the importance of the individual in health should not be taken as an argument for neglecting the effects of working conditions, of housing and of marketing food, tobacco and alcohol."

A definite note of disapproval of the feckless is also beginning to creep into official pronouncements. The current Government's most recent statement on health policy, *Care in Action*[8] begins its chapter on prevention:

"The prevention of mental and physical ill health is a prime objective and an area in which the individual has clear responsibilities. No-one can wholly escape illness or injury but there are plenty of risks to health which are within the individual's power to reduce or avoid. *Too many endanger their health through ignorance and social pressures.*" (my italics)

This kind of statement embodies a subtle change in the self help philosophy. Now it is not just that people could be healthier if they looked after themselves better, but that people get ill through being anti-social and irresponsible. In a few deft logical steps what the ill health working class people struggle against has been rendered a product of their own inadequacies. They have only themselves to blame. The Government, employers, polluters, food and tobacco manufacturers and all those who profit from our ill health are at a stroke absolved.

When you think about it class inequalities in health are an indictment of our whole society: economic priorities, the organisation of work, social priorities, the organisation of domestic life, planning, housing and environmental policies. Telling us we should be looking after ourselves distracts us from this reality. When the 'look after yourself' thinking becomes embodied in the everyday practices of health professionals, it is part of the process by which the social order which destroys our health is reproduced.

This is why the self-help message is an anti-health message.

TOWARDS AN ALTERNATIVE STRATEGY FOR PREVENTION

BUT to reject the self-help message does not imply a return to confidence in the wonders of medicine. What is needed is an alternative strategy for prevention which takes account of both the class origins of ill health and lay people's growing interest in taking more control over their own health.

Such a strategy would be based on four basic principles:

(a) *Hard information not 'do's and don'ts'*
Health education should be less a matter of telling people what to do, than giving them the information on which to make their own choices. Lay people do not want 'do's and don'ts', but hard information about their own bodies. People want to know what a fallopian tube is, what the difference is between arthritis and rheumatism, what is in the food they are eating, where cancer comes from and whether it can be cured. They are hungry for information and want straight answers.

(b) *Building a new health common sense*
Current levels of understanding of health and illness are poor. Most people have been told that ill health is caused by germs. They have not been educated to look at their own life experience to discover what is causing their asthma, dermatitis or back pain. Medicine has tended to discourage people from valuing their own insights about their personal health. What we want is to

create a new popular understanding of health and illness, so that just as it is now automatic for people to wash their hands when they have been to the toilet, it would be automatic to think: what additives are there in the food I am eating? Will the new productivity deal the management want to bring in affect the stress we work under? How will the plan to reroute the traffic in our area affect the lead in the air?

At one level people know what is making them ill. They know they are under stress, or the house is damp or their work makes them overtired, but by victim blaming and focusing on cure rather than causes, current medical practice has tended to undermine rather than endorse these insights. What we need is to help create a new kind of health common sense so that it becomes a second nature for people to reflect on how their lives and their environment affect their health.

(c) *Support for collective action*
Although individuals are often powerless on their own to affect what is making them ill, there are many possibilities for change through collective action. One of the most powerful lessons the women's movement has learned is that sharing your problems with others can give you strength to struggle against difficulties in your own life. One of the central ideas in the trade union movement is that through collective action and solidarity living standards and working conditions can be improved. The struggle for better health involves a combination of these two principles. Health workers have a role to play supporting collective discussion of common health problems and collective action to improve living and working conditions. This may mean helping a tenants association do a survey of the health of people with bad housing, or helping a local shop stewards committee by finding out for them the dangers of the substances they work with, or encouraging women with depression to meet and talk.

(d) *Challenging the existing economic order*
Recognising that ill health is a reflection of the material conditions within which people live and work, prevention is about changing these conditions. A far reaching transformation of social and economic organisation is needed if inequalities in health are to be reduced. This may mean challenging relationships of control and domination in our society.

Although health workers may not necessarily be able to deliver miracle cures, they play a vital role in people's understanding or misunderstanding of what is making them ill and how ill health can be prevented. There is no neutrality. All the time in everyday encounters with the public they are shaping how people see their health and what they do about it. Doctors, health educators and other health care workers who reject the assumptions of those who blame life style for ill health and want to see an alternative approach to prevention, should perhaps examine their own practice to see how they could better encourage rather than undermine understanding of and action on the social and economic roots of ill health. Some questions we could ask ourselves are:

* Am I involved in encouraging people to feel guilty or helping them take control over their own health?
* Am I helping my patients or clients understand the preventable nature of ill health and its social and economic origins?
* Am I involved in helping them understand their own bodies and illnesses, or am I mystifying them?
* Am I listening to my patients talk about their life experience and involved in helping them identify and understand the health problems they face?
* Am I helping patients with common problems (for instance those isolated in the home or working in the same factory) to link up with each other?
* Is my medical records system designed to help identify the environmental causes of common problems my patients face?
* What collective action on health issues could I give practical support to?

What the Government booklets leave out when they talk about how health in the nineteenth century was improved through better living standards, is that many of these improvements were gained through bitter struggle, in which working class people banded together in trade unions and political organisations to fight collectively for change. This principle holds goods today. It is through tenants associations fighting for rehousing, through trade unions fighting for better working conditions, through pensioners fighting for better pensions that the hope for better health lies. There are no short cuts. Fighting for better health means confronting employers like British Leyland, who speed up the production line so fast that many workers have nervous breakdowns. It means challenging a form of social organisation in which women are isolated in the home. It means taking on an economic system which depends on the production of health destructive products, puts workers lives at risk and leaves three million people on the dole. Health workers can make their contribution to this struggle in all kinds of ways. Challenging the idea that looking after ourselves is an individual responsibility and fostering a new approach to prevention which speaks to rather than denies people's class experience is one urgent and crucial task.

REFERENCES
[1] HMSO (1977) *First Report from the Expenditure Committee Session 1976/77, Preventive Medicine, Volume 1.*
[2] Department of Health and Social Security (1976) *Prevention and Health: Everybody's Business.*
[3] HMSO: (1977) *Prevention and Health.*
[4] Department of Health and Social Security (1976) *Prevention and Health: Everybody's Business.*
[5] ibid.
[6] *Avoiding Heart Attacks*, HMSO 1981.
[7] Self Care — Self Blame, *Lancet* Vol II for 1981, No. 8251, 17 October pp 846-847.
[8] Department of Health and Social Security: *Care in Action: A Handbook of policies and priorities for the Health and Social Services*, February 1981.

* Note: Inequalities in Health is no longer available from the Department of Health, as only a few hundred copies were printed. A useful summary, *The Unequal Health of the Nation*, is available from the Trades Union Congress.

Health Education: prevention or subversion?

B. K. TONES, M.A., M.Sc., Ph.D.
Principal Lecturer in Health Education, Leeds Polytechnic, Health Education Unit, Hollin Hall, Hollin Road, Leeds LS16 5JR

IT IS no easy task to provide a concise yet illuminating definition of health education. In fact it is tempting to follow the example of the psychologist who defined intelligence as what intelligence tests measure, and say that health education is what health educators do. It is, however, possible to identify different philosophical approaches to the practice of health education and in this paper four such approaches will be examined.

THE 'EDUCATIONAL' APPROACH

THOSE WHO adopt an 'educational' stance — consciously or unconsciously — are likely to do so either because they have a rather naive understanding of the dynamics of health-related behaviour or because they believe it is unethical to use persuasion or other forms of coercion to motivate individuals to adopt a healthy life style. The Society of Public Health Educators of America, in formulating its code of ethical practice, emphasised the principle of voluntariness.

"Health Educators value privacy, dignity, and the worth of the individual . . . Health Educators observe the principle of informed consent . . . Health Educators support change by choice, not coercion."[1]

The principle of informed choice does not, of course, mean that the client is merely offered information about health risks and then left to make up his own mind about whether or not to take any notice of the facts provided. Sound educational practice would involve ensuring that any health information had been understood. The educationist would then arrange for clients to share and explore their beliefs and values in relation to the health information and discuss its implications for action. For example, school children might be presented with facts about family planning and unwanted pregnancies and then be asked to discuss the implications of not using contraceptives for their own well-being, the well-being of their partners and the health of the unwanted baby. Similarly, women attending ante-natal classes who had been provided with information listing the benefits of breast-feeding might subsequently explore with other women in the group the implications for them of choosing one or other form of feeding and discuss their anxieties and uncertainties.

In some educational contexts, the client might be given the opportunity to practise making decisions. For instance, a group of adolescents in school might be asked to role play a scene in a disco and try to handle a situation in which they were offered drugs. The difficulties of resisting peer pressures might then be discussed in the ensuing de-briefing session. The main elements in this 'educational' approach could be expressed diagrammatically as follows.

Fig. 1

It is worth noting in passing that evaluation of the effectiveness of the educational approach merely involves demonstrating that the client has a genuine understanding of the situation. No attempt would be made to devise attitude-change measures or look for 'healthy' behavioural outcomes.

In many ways the educational approach is an attractive proposition for the health educator. Providing information and promoting understanding is undoubtedly an easier task than changing well-established and often pleasurable behaviours. Moreover, he may congratulate himself on having adopted an ethical stance in avoiding persuasion and propaganda. However, in adopting this approach it is easy to overlook the fact that many people are in no position to use the information provided and make an 'informed choice'. For many individuals the options are limited or non-existent. The middle class male who has elected to stop smoking is in a very different position from the highly stressed, social class V housewife who exists in squalid circumstances and for whom a cigarette represents a rare and fleeting moment of nirvana. Equally, in a community having a predominance of unskilled manual workers where the prevalence of smoking by males will be of the order of 60 per cent, children could not be said to have the same degree of choice as those who have been raised in a middle class environment where only 25 per cent of males are likely to be smokers.[2] Middle class parents, in addition to providing a non-smoking model, are also likely to provide a socialising experience which predisposes their children to value the deferring of present pleasure for some future reward (pay now; live later — and longer!), which builds into them a belief in their own autonomy and power to control their destiny, and which at the same time provides them with high self esteem and self respect. Such children are much more likely to resist unhealthy pressures and adopt healthy life styles.

McKeown[3] illustrates the illusory nature of freedom of choice in relation to recruitment to smoking.

"Our habits commonly begin as pleasures of which we have no need and end as necessities in which we have no pleasure. Nevertheless we tend to resent the suggestion that anyone should try to change them, even on the disarming grounds that they do so for our

R.S.H. 3 1981   B. K. TONES

own good . . . it is said that the individual must be free to choose whether he wishes to smoke. But he is not free; with a drug of addiction the option is open only at the beginning, so that the critical decision to smoke is taken, not by consenting adults but by children below the age of consent."

One might argue that if people do not have equal access to informed decision-making, it is unethical not to intervene. For example, McKeown goes on to ask whether it is acceptable to ". . . induce children to become addicts at an age when they neither know nor much care about the associated risks". The need to persuade and motivate people to modify their behaviour for their own good rather than merely offer them a choice underlies the preventive approach to health education.

THE PREVENTIVE APPROACH

PREVENTIVE HEALTH education is perhaps the best known approach and operates within the context of medical care. It is based on assumptions that not only is prevention better than cure, but that curative medicine is failing to deal with contemporary community health problems. A further assumption is that since behaviour is involved in the aetiology of modern disease, prevention is best achieved by prescribing health education in order to modify the behaviours which are responsible for the disease. It is worth examining these assumptions in more detail.

It is generally accepted by epidemiologists that major improvements in community health have had little, if anything, to do with medicine until the second quarter of the twentieth century. The factors responsible for the major improvements which occurred in health during this period have been social, behavioural and environmental. More particularly, improved nutritional status has been identified as a key determinant of health and this has in turn derived from a combination of improved food supply and population control. Sanitary measures — the provision of pure drinking water and sewage disposal — were also of paramount importance. The development of effective therapeutic measures — the 'magic bullets' — came rather too late to have had any major effect on the infectious diseases which were largely responsible for mortality. With the demise of the infectious diseases, chronic degenerative disorders — heart disease and the cancers for example — came into prominence and curative medicine has had relatively little success with these. The relative ineffectiveness of coronary care units[4][5] serves to underline not only the limitations of high technology medicine, but emphasises its increasing cost. Cochrane[6] strikingly illustrates what he called the input-output gap between expenditure on the N.H.S. and the benefits derived from this expenditure with his parable of the crematorium worker.

"I once asked a worker at a crematorium, who had a curiously contented look on his face, what he found so satisfying about his work. He replied that what fascinated him was the way in which so much went in and so little came out. I thought of advising him to get a job in the National Health Service."

When considering the input-output equation we should perhaps note in passing that high technology has its iatrogenic side effects — a point made quite forcibly by Asimov:

"In 1976 the doctors of Los Angeles went on strike for five weeks abandoning their patients to the mercy of natural recovery. The weekly death rate in Los Angeles promptly dropped from 19·8 deaths per 100,000 to an average of 16·2 per 100,000 during the strike-bound five weeks. When the doctors went busily back to their stethoscopes and tongue depressors, the weekly death rate promptly jumped to an average of 20·4 per 100,000 over the next five weeks."

(Asimov, I.: Omni, January, 1979)

A second assumption underlying the preventive approach is that behaviour plays a significant part in the aetiology of chronic degenerative diseases. The importance of such factors as diet, lack of exercise and smoking has been well documented. In fact, it would appear that the adoption of the life style of such sects as Mormons or Seventh Day Adventists is tantamount to a guarantee of several extra years of higher quality living.[7][8] If people can be persuaded to adopt and sustain healthy practices then the 'diseases of affluence' might be prevented and history might be repeated — as McKeown[3] asserts:

"Past improvement has been due to mainly modification of behaviour and changes in the environment and it is to these same influences that we must look particularly for further advance."

Health Education, then, is concerned to prevent disease and disability by modifying behaviour — by developing new 'healthy' behaviours and changing existing 'unhealthy' practices. It is customary to describe different stages of prevention and it is equally valid to categorise preventive health education in terms of primary, secondary and tertiary stages. Table I below shows the relationship between these categories and the standard sociological descriptions of role-related behaviour.

The term 'health behaviour' describes any activity undertaken by an individual who believes he is healthy in order to prevent future illness or detect it in an asymptomatic state. 'Illness behaviour' refers to behaviours adopted by an individual who experiences symptoms in order to decide whether or not he is really ill and, if so, what to do about it. 'Sick role behaviour' occurs when an individual has decided he is ill, has sought medical advice and the doctor has confirmed his illness. It involves assuming the rights and duties of the patient — including exemption from work and agreeing to comply with medical advice. It can be seen from Table I that one commonly accepted function of preventive health education is to promote the development and proper use of medical services and this may happen at either primary, secondary or tertiary levels.

The influence of social and psychological factors on illness behaviour cannot be over-stated. Anyone assuming that symptom experience is related in any simple way to a 'rational' use of medical services should note the following principles derived from research findings on utilisation of G.P. services:

(a) A majority of individuals have experienced distressing symptoms in recent time.
(b) A relatively small proportion seek medical advice.
(c) Consultation is not related in any simple way to symptom seriousness.
(d) Doctors, patients and patients' relatives may all perceive symptom seriousness differently.
(e) Those patients who do consult may present only a few of their symptoms — and not necessarily the most serious or worrying.
(f) The presentation of symptoms may be an excuse for counselling of a general nature.

A fair proportion of patients will be dissatisfied with the consultation; they may not understand what the doctor has said; they are likely to forget a substantial proportion of what they have been told. On average 50

HEALTH EDUCATION

TABLE I

Stage of Prevention	Role-Related Behaviour	Type of Health Education
PRIMARY Preventing onset of disease or detecting it in asymptomatic stage	HEALTH BEHAVIOUR	PRIMARY HEALTH EDUCATION: e.g. Smoking cessation; acceptance of immunisation; hygienic practices; utilising cervical cytology services
SECONDARY Preventing development of disease and reversing process where possible	ILLNESS BEHAVIOUR	SECONDARY HEALTH EDUCATION: e.g. Compliance with hypertensive therapy; seeking early diagnosis for potentially threatening symptoms such as 7 warning signs of cancer Appropriate utilisation of GP service
TERTIARY Rehabilitation Resuming as full a life as possible despite residual impairment from disease Accepting impending death	SICK ROLE BEHAVIOUR	TERTIARY HEALTH EDUCATION: e.g. Compliance with therapy Accepting 'healthy status' and abandoning 'sick role' Accepting dentures

per cent of patients will fail to comply with the medical advice provided.

Tertiary prevention is, like its counterpart in clinical medicine, a relatively neglected function lacking in glamour and prestige. It is worth quoting McKeown's observation about the importance of care.[3]

". . . since most major disease and disabilities are either preventible or intractible, care rather than cure should be our concept of the main focus of medical attention."

It may serve to emphasise the importance of tertiary prevention if we repeat Ashley and Klein's[9] estimate that at present trends, by 1992, 75·5 per cent of hospital beds for men and 93·7 per cent of non-maternity beds for women will be filled by patients over the age of 65. We might also add that 50 per cent of the elderly report some disability[10] and the average cost of treating people who are over 75 is seven times the cost of treating people of working age.[10]

THE RADICAL APPROACH

THE FACT that health education has apparently focussed on the preventive approach at the expense of alternatives has been a source of some concern. For instance, Hannu Vuori, Regional Officer for Primary Health Care, W.H.O., has lamented the apparent subservience of health education to the medical model.[11] There is an increasing interest in what is here referred to as a radical approach to health education, that is an approach which seeks the roots of health problems and finds them in social, economic and political factors. McKinlay[12] dramatically underlines the dangers of reacting to the superficial aspects of illness manifestation when he describes the continuous and frustrating process of dragging a succession of drowning victims from a fast flowing river and hastily applying artificial respiration.

"Again and again, without end, goes the sequence. You know, I am so busy jumping in, pulling them to shore, applying artificial respiration, that I have no time to see who the hell is upstream pushing them all in."

When we follow McKinlay's advice and 'refocus upstream', we find at source major social correlates of ill health such as poverty and disadvantage. It is an acknowledged and chastening fact that there is as big a gap between the health of social classes I and V today

as there was thirty years ago. And this applies to virtually all diseases. Would it not then seem more sensible to try to deal with poverty than to persuade individual members of disadvantaged groups to alter their life style? The economic basis of health needs little elaboration: it might be argued with some justification that if government was really concerned to make some inroad into the tobacco-induced epidemic of disease, it would not be so concerned to avoid alienating the tobacco manufacturers and to safeguard its tax revenues. It might be argued that instead of advising individuals to adopt a prudent diet[13] D.H.S.S. might have done better to influence government fiscal policy to ensure that products high in dietary fibre and low in saturated fat were both readily accessible and cheap. Indeed, the pamphlet, 'Food and Profit'[14] argues that ill health is socially rather than individually produced and asserts that

". . . the major force responsible for the social production of an unhealthy diet is the drive of the food industry to accumulate profits, personal choice . . . is seriously limited."

Vincente Navarro[15] claims that the 'victim-blaming' approach of preventive health education is acceptable to a profit-seeking, capitalist society since it poses no real threat to the social system

". . . rather than weakening, it strengthens the basic tenets of bourgeois individualism . . . far from being a threat to the power structure, this life-style politics complements and is easily co-optable by the controllers of the system."

Draper's[16] detailed and comprehensive analysis of the ways in which the current pursuit of productivity and economic growth is damaging to mental, physical and social health makes a similar point. Even the least politically orientated observer cannot fail to recognise the implications for all aspects of community and individual health of unemployment and what Toffler[17] called 'future shock'.

It will be clear from what has been said so far that a major task of radical health education is to generate public awareness and concern in relation to the kind of issue described above. Since knowledge alone is insufficient for action perhaps the radical approach has, in common with preventive health education, a need to resort to persuasive tactics if community action is to result.

R.S.H. 3 1981   *B. K. TONES*

AN APPROACH TO SELF EMPOWERMENT

FROM WHAT has been said so far it would appear that health educators are faced with a dilemma. If they adopt an educational approach they might have to accept a role which involves the provision of good advice which will subsequently be ignored! Yet if they adopt a preventive approach they might have to resort to 'unethical' coercion and act as handmaidens to the medical model. On the other hand, the promotion of major social, political and economic change would appear a mammoth task involving either ineffectual posturing or commitment to degrees of subversive action. There may, however, be an alternative approach — an approach involving the pursuit of 'self empowerment'. The aim of such an approach would be to facilitate the kind of informed choice which was earlier considered an illusory goal. Four strategies would be involved. One of these would aim to promote beliefs and attitudes favourable to deferring present immediate reward for some future more substantial benefit — for instance, abandoning over-eating for a promise of a healthier and longer middle and old age. A second strategy would attempt to increase 'internal locus of control',[18] in other words would challenge beliefs that life and health were controlled by fate or powerful people. This strategy would be complemented by an endeavour to enhance individual self esteem: an individual who values and respects himself is not only more likely to respond to an educational approach showing how to safeguard health, but will be more able to resist the various pressures which lead to unhealthy practices. It might, of course, be argued — and with some justification — that even a self empowered individual would be unable to have any impact on adverse social conditions and an oppressive environment. This may be true. However, the development of certain social skills — for example, assertiveness training — might enable the individual to challenge his environment and at the same time provide him with an experience of success which enhances self esteem and increases his belief in his capacity to control his life.

It is difficult to see how the development of a deferred gratification value might be achieved — except through patient attempts to teach parents and future parents how to rear their children — perhaps in the context of parentcraft and child care courses in schools. However, there are already detailed programmes of health education designed to promote self esteem and to equip children with various life skills.[19] [20] [21] For instance, Hopson and Scally[20] provide teaching programmes designed to develop 'life skills' such as the following:

How to communicate effectively
How to manage time effectively
How to cope with unemployment
How to be assertive
How to work in groups
How to be positive about oneself

It would be naive to assume that such programmes will find ready acceptance in schools, but there are signs of increasing awareness of the importance of promoting personal and social development in school children. It is also worth acknowledging the increasing number of community development projects orientated towards health and having implicit or explicit self empowerment aims.[22]

Four approaches to health education have been separately identified in this paper. They need not be separate and although they frequently represent different philosophical standpoints they often overlap in practice and coexist more or less happily.

REFERENCES

1. Society for Public Health Education. *Code of Ethics*. October 15, 1976. San Francisco, California.
2. OPCS Monitor GHS 79/2.
3. McKEOWN, T. (1976) *The Role of Medicine: Dream, Mirage or Nemesis?* Nuffield Provincial Hospitals Trust: London.
4. MATHER, H. G. et al (1971) "Acute myocardial infarction: home and hospital treatment." *British Medical Journal*, vol. 3, 334-338.
5. COLLING, A. et al (1976) "Teesside coronary survey: an epidemiological study of acute attacks of myocardial infarction." *British Medical Journal*, vol. 2, 1169.
6. COCHRANE, A. L. (1971) *Effectiveness and efficiency: random reflections on the health service*. Nuffield Provincial Hospitals Trust: London.
7. BRESLOW, L. "A Quantitative Approach to the World Health Organization Definition of Health." *International Journal of Epidemiology*, vol. 1, no. 4, Winter 1972, 347-55.
   BELLOC, N. B. and BRESLOW, L. "Relationship of Physical Health Status and Health Practices." *Preventive Medicine*, vol. 1, no. 3, August 1972, 409-21.
   BELLOC, N. B. "Relationship of Health Practices and Mortality." *Preventive Medicine*, vol. 2, 1973, 67-81.
8. KRISTEIN, M. M. et al (1977) "Health Economics and Preventive Care." *Science*, vol. 195, 457-462.
9. KLEIN, R. and ASHLEY, J. (1972) "Old-Age Health." *New Society*, Jan. 6, 13-15.
10. HARRIS, A. (1968) *Social welfare for the elderly*. London: H.M.S.O.
11. VUORI, H. (1980) "The medical model and the objectives of health education." *International Journal of Health Education*, vol. XXIII, no. 1, 1-8.
12. McKINLAY, J. B. (1975) "A case for refocussing upstream — the political economy of illness." In *Applying Behavioural Science to Cardiovascular Risk* (occasional paper).
13. D.H.S.S. (1978) *Eating for Health*. H.M.S.O.
14. *Food and Profit*. The Politics of Health Group. Pamphlet No. One.
15. NAVARRO, V. (1976) "The underdevelopment of health of working America: causes, consequences, and possible solutions." *American Journal of Public Health*, vol. 66, 538-547.
16. DRAPER, P. (1977) "Health and Wealth." *Royal Society of Health Journal*, June 1977.
17. TOFFLER, A. (1970). *Future Shock*. Pan: London.
18. "Health Locus of Control." *Health Education Monographs*, vol. 6, no. 2, Spring 1978.
19. Schools Council Health Education Project 5-13. *All About Me* and *Think Well*. Nelson.
20. HOPSON, B. and SCALLY, M. (1980) *Lifeskills Teaching Programmes*. Lifeskills Associates: Leeds.
21. BALDWIN, J. and WELLS, H. (1980) *Active Tutorial Work*. Blackwell.
22. HUBLEY, J. (1980) *Community Health Projects in London*. Report on a study tour.

In practice

HEALTH PROFILE

Every picture tells the story

In a unique approach to community health profiling, Plymouth health visitor Joy Harrison used photographs to illustrate her study of the problems faced by residents of just one street in a particularly deprived housing estate on her patch.

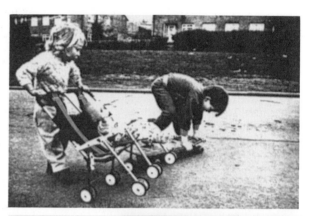

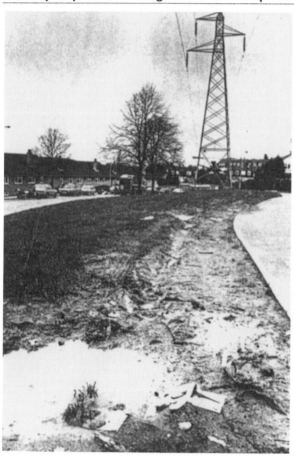

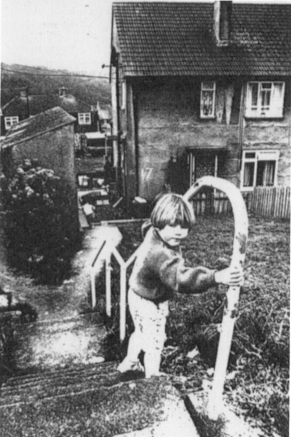

A central strip of muddy grass divides the houses on the north and south sides of the street. A high-power electricity pylon stands in the middle of the central green. Children as young as seven have been seen climbing right to the top of the pylon. The local electricity company has fitted additional safety barriers – but turned down a request for funding towards a play park. One of the residents now keeps a watch for children on the pylon. Some are worried about other health risks from the pylon. One resident commented: 'The housing department said if you can prove there is a risk of cancer living near a pylon, then we will move you'.

With nowhere else to go, children playing on the street are at risk from speeding cars. 'Some people are just idiots. Visitors don't realise how many kiddies there are down here. How a kid hasn't been killed is a miracle', one resident said. The nearest play park is run-down and unsafe for children under five. Another resident said 'Give us the materials and the men in the street will build our own'

The ground-floor flats on the south side are below street level, with steep front gardens and concrete steps up to the road. Residents are forced to keep the lights on all year round as the living rooms receive no direct natural light. Overcrowding is a major problem. Some families on the south side have four or five children. Children on access visits at weekends create further accommodation problems. Families are desperate to be rehoused.

Only the ground floor flats have locks on their windows – to keep burglars out. Upstairs the windows can be easily opened, creating a major hazard for small children. It would cost £40 to put locks on the windows: a sum beyond the resources of most families

In practice

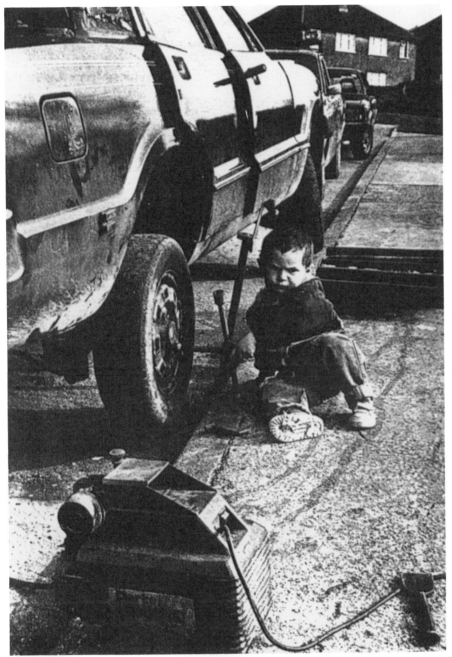

Lewes Gardens is a cul-de-sac on the Whitleigh housing estate in Plymouth. Forty two-bedroom maisonettes house 65 adults and 69 children; 49 of the children are under five. The estate was built hurriedly in the early 1950s to replace bombed houses in the city and the housing is of poor quality. There is a high level of unemployment; most families are dependent on state benefits.

'This report was not intended as a sophisticated, scientific report. It demonstrates what most of us are aware of but few will face up to: that many people in our community are living in unhealthy, inadequate circumstances – in most cases through no fault of their own', says Dr Noel Olsen, director of public health for Plymouth and Torbay health authority.

Asked if they would be prepared to come to a residents' meeting to discuss how to get improvements on the estate. 23 adults out of 21 households said yes, and 18 were willing to serve on a committee.

The project was funded by Plymouth and Torbay health authority public health department. The photographs were taken by Paul Courtney, Plymouth and Torbay health authority public relations officer.

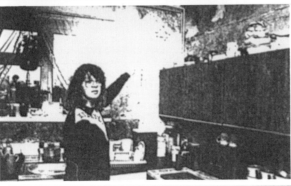

The houses are badly-designed and prone to cold and damp. Every flat suffers from condensation. The wallpaper in newly-decorated rooms can peel off after a couple of months, causing heartbreak to many of the low income families who have spent precious resources on creating a home. The damp and condensation causes clothing to turn mouldy in cupboards and wardrobes, and furniture and fittings to turn black. Central heating is being installed – rents have gone up by £5 a week to cover the costs – but, with VAT on fuel, residents may not be able to afford to use it. Similar systems installed elsewhere in the area are said to cost £25 a week to run. One young mother was spending £12 a week on coal out of her weekly benefit as a single parent with four children to feed and clothe. She could only afford one 25lb bag at a time, carried home from the shops on the baby's buggy. Eight out of 44 children were reported asthmatic and requiring medication, and 15 were said to be 'chesty', and to suffer frequent coughs and colds

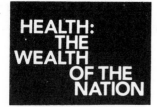

Community mothers: trick or treat?

To many health visitors they are a threat. To others they are a unique and invaluable resource. CATH JACKSON talks to the health visitors and women involved in two projects pioneering community mother programmes in England. *Health visitor 1992; 65, 6: 199-201*

'I don't claim to know all the answers and I do ask for help from the health visitors. But working together I feel we can help more people than just health visitors on their own.'

Donna is a 'community mother', one of five local women working with health visitors in Tilbury, Essex, to support families with young children. Forty families are receiving the kind of 'workaday' support that in a better world mothers, grandmothers, the woman next door, would have provided. The difference is that Donna is part of an organised programme, an NHS service funded by Basildon and Thurrock health authority, and she is paid for her time and expenses.

'Some families don't welcome health visitors easily; they see them as "the enemy". Some families accept me easier because, as one of my mums said: "I like you Donna because you're just like me — dead common",' Donna believes.

'Community care for women should be in the community', says Rashida Riaz, one of 25 Asian women involved in the Nottingham Asian community mothers' programme. She believes she can help bridge the language and cultural divide between the predominantly white, western health visitors and women from the large Asian community in Nottingham City sector. 'I understand what they are telling me. They don't have to explain themselves the whole time.'

Their comments sum up the argument behind Dr Walter Barker's controversial 'community mothers' project, part of the childhood development programme he has pioneered with a five-strong team in Bristol for the past 13 years.

Tilbury launched its community mothers programme with the backing of Basildon and Thurrock community services managers just over a year ago.

One part time health visitor was already using the child development programme with all the first time mothers in Tilbury. She is now developing her role as the community mother trainer as well. The one full time health visitor and two other part-timers provide the routine child health service. Another part timer, Celia Suppiah, is the family support visitor for families with acute coping problems and also supports and co-ordinates the community mothers team.

The community mothers programme has to be built on an established first-parent visiting programme, Celia Suppiah stresses. The community mothers work to the same principles of 'empowerment', using the same simple, cartoon-illustrated materials developed by Walter Barker's team to boost women's confidence in their own child-rearing abilities.

Walter Barker's team help select and train women whom the health visitors have recommended. The community mothers meet monthly to discuss their work and talk over any problems they have encountered. Celia Suppiah also visits each community mother at their home every two months to talk individually.

The families receiving visits from community mothers are those with more than one child who, while not experiencing acute difficulties, would in the view of their health visitor benefit from extra ongoing support.

'People who are up to their eye-balls in trouble get all the help that's going', Donna says. 'People with "small problems" would also fall into that big hole if left without any help and then they'd need a JCB to dig them out.

'We're giving the people with the small problems a little shovel and forget about the JCB.'

The health visitors asked local women how they would feel about receiving visits from a community mother before the scheme was launched. 'Many said they would have liked to have been able to talk to another mother rather than bother the health visitor', Celia Suppiah says.

Training

The community mothers have clear guidelines on the limits of their responsibilities. 'We train them to encourage mothers to come up with their own ideas and to discourage dependence. That's why they only visit once a month. They work with the mothers only, not the children, and they don't give health advice.' If a problem emerges outside the community mother's remit, she will refer it to the family's health visitor, who maintains overall responsibility for the family.

But the health visitor is only brought in with the family's agreement, Celia Suppiah stresses. She agrees it is difficult to 'draw the line' between a problem which can be tackled with the support of the community mother and more complex problems which require health visitor intervention. Not infrequently mothers reveal problems to the community mother that they have felt unable to share with the health visitor.

But the community mothers are not expected to report back every problem to the health visitors, Celia Suppiah stresses. 'She would lose credibility in the community and with the mother.'

It's a question of 'creating their own balance' between friend and sympathetic supporter and representative of the official health services. There are, however, clear guidelines in situations where a community mother becomes aware of, or is told of, harm being done to a child. She will discuss the situation confidentially with the co-ordinator, who will then take it further if necessary. So far there has been only one such case and the mother willingly agreed for the health visitor to come in and support her.

Close friendship may develop between a community mother and her 'client' family, but 'we would worry if they were spending a lot of time with a lot of their families. They may lose objectivity', Celia Suppiah points out.

There have been no problems with 'over-involvement' or dependency; no crisis calls to health visitors in the dead of night, although the community mothers have the health visitors' home telephone numbers. Celia Suppiah suggests that support from the community mothers does, in fact, help diffuse such family crises before they explode.

Bridging the gap

The Nottingham programme follows a slightly different pattern in that it aims to offer a community mother to all mothers in the city's Asian community for whom English is not the first language. It also operates at arm's length from the health visiting service.

The programme developed gradually, in fits and starts, from a growing recognition that the routine health visiting service was failing to meet the needs of Asian women, largely because of the language and cultural divide.

'This was the early 80s. When we asked for money for interpreters we were told it wasn't necessary; that the Asian community would provide volunteers. We were using a clerical assistant as an interpreter because there was nothing else',

In practice

explains Barbara Lymn, recently retired as manager of ethnic services in Nottingham City sector.

There was a high turnover among health visitors. 'We were trying to find ways to address what the health visitors were telling us: that they didn't know what the needs of the Asian families were; didn't feel they were giving a good service.'

Sneh Kashyap, now full-time co-ordinator of the community mothers programme, was originally employed part-time as an interpreter in June 1990. In

receive inappropriate advice or stay away for fear that their needs will not be respected or understood.

Women who can speak English often don't feel confident enough to assert their needs with white British medical and health professionals. Sneh Kashyap recalls how her first baby was taken from her in hospital and given a bottle — this was back in the early 80s — even though she wanted, and the Asian tradition is, to breastfeed.

Asian women, told by the health visitor that spicey food

'I had been at home bringing up my children for five years. I really needed to get out. It's brought me confidence. Being at home with the children, you think that's it. But there is life after having children', Rashida Riaz says.

As in Tilbury, the community mothers receive initial training and ongoing support from both Walter Barker's team and from the Nottingham health visiting service. Ongoing training sessions cover topics like breast feeding and weaning, immunisation, health

community mothers visiting a family on her caseload. The health visitors continue to visit and the mothers are encouraged to come to clinic and use the routine child health services. The health visitors 'watched their families closely' at first, but are now completely accepting of the programme, Sneh reports. She now wants to develop closer links with the midwives.

Kate Billingham, professional development manager for Nottingham community nursing services, recently took over management of the programme from Barbara Lymn. She believes that the service should have been allowed to develop in a 'protected' environment. 'It needed space to develop its own character and not be "professionalised".'

Now, however, she would like to see a gradual move to closer working. 'At the end of the day it is not a separate thing. It is part of the primary care service — and health visitors can learn such a lot from it.' There is, she believes, a role for health visitors as 'supporters'; part of their wider public health and community development remit.

Only one woman has been 'counselled out' of the Nottingham programme. The 25 women involved come from the three main sikh, muslim and hindu communities in the city and between them speak all the Asian dialects. It is vital that the programme should be accepted by the Asian communities: all the community mothers wear Asian dress when visiting families; 'If they are strict muslims I will wear a head scarf as well', Rashida Riaz says. Walter Barker was asked to speak to the men of the community. 'They all accepted it with open arms. They were really pleased that there was now something like this for their women', Sneh Kashyap reports.

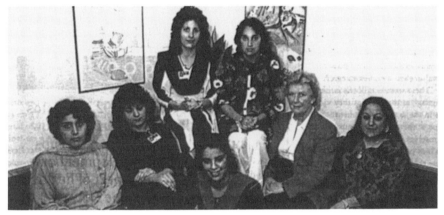

Nottingham community mothers: 'time to build closer links with health visitors'

photo: John Birdsall

November 1990 the health authority agreed to put up £20,000 to launch a community mothers programme for Asian families. Sneh Kashyap and two others — who later dropped out — received training in first-parent visiting (Nottingham too has a first-parent visiting programme) and worked for year with ten families to pilot the project. The first community mothers were recruited in November 1991 and there are now 25, covering 90 per cent of the target client group.

The Asian 'joint family system' is an important source of support for young Asian mothers but it can also create problems. When a woman marries she joins her husband's family, where the mother-in-law runs the household and has a central role in bringing up the children, Sneh Kashyap explains. But the young mother can lose confidence and self-esteem and feel undermined and unsupported. Opportunity to talk with another woman from their community helps rebuild their enjoyment in their children.

Language difficulties mean that Asian women may miss out on health services available to them,

should not be given to babies and unable to find vegetarian packaged foods, weaned their children on the sweetened desserts, creating a problem with tooth decay.

'These issues weren't recognised because of the language and cultural barriers. Women felt ashamed to explain to the health visitor that they were vegetarian; they felt it was a sign of poverty', Sneh Kashyap believes. 'We all thought the health visitor knew best.'

Women are recruited to the programme through Asian women's community groups and by word of mouth.

Rashida Riaz was recommended by her health visitor and interviewed in her home by Sneh Kashyap. Sneh looks for personal experience of mothering, for language skills and for commitment — 'how much they are going to put into the work; how she feels about working for the community. It shouldn't be "What am I going to get out of it"; I'm looking for give, not take', she stresses.

The community mothers themselves benefit from the training and work.

records and family planning.

The community mothers may not give direct advice on these issues to families, but 'we realised it would help their confidence if they knew about certain basic health subjects', Barbara Lymn explains.

Working together

In Nottingham, the community mothers take referrals from health visitors but operate as a separate entity, with Sneh Kashyap liaising between them.

'At the start we felt that the community mothers should report directly to a health visitor, but we realised this might injure the programme if the health visitors were seen to be "in control"', Barbara Lymn says. 'There was a danger that we would fall into the trap where the health visitor dictated the programme, rather than the programme being offered to women who wanted it.'

Monthly 'coffee mornings' are held with the health visitors and Sneh Kashyap reports directly to the health visitor responsible any problems encountered by the

Inside and out

There are contrasting views on the implications for confidentiality if, as Walter Barker believes, the community mothers visit locally to their homes. 'My next door neighbour wouldn't want me to know her private business', Sneh Kashyap believes.

Walter Barker stresses the principles of community self-help and 'empowerment'. 'If the community mother comes from

In practice

outside, it is saying to the community that it does not have the resources to help itself, that it still needs "outside" support.'

Rashida Riaz visits families local to her own home in Nottingham and has not found it a problem. 'I hope I have established a reputation locally for being trustworthy. My main fear was that women would not like to meet me on the street corner; they'd be thinking "Here comes bossy boots".' It is a new challenge with every new family, she says. Celia Suppiah says that any anxiety among families receiving visits from a local community mother soon vanishes and there is no evidence that trust or confidentiality is abused. Every community mother signs a confidentiality form before starting visiting.

Pay is another tricky issue. In Nottingham the women are paid £2.50 an hour; Walter Barker says £3.00 should be the maximum. 'It is not meant to be a paid job with a contract', Celia Suppiah emphasises. 'It's an informal community network, voluntary work really with expenses paid to cover travel and childcare.' Many of the community mothers are on state benefits and might lose out if they were paid any more.

But in Nottingham it is seen a important that the women are paid; their status with the community — and within their families — would be undermined if they were seen as 'volunteers', Sneh Kashyap says. 'The husbands say, "Well, where is the money?"'

The Nottingham community mothers have discussed increasing the hourly rate. 'I wouldn't want women to move on just because the pay is bad', Sneh Kashyap says. She hopes to get money to employ one of the women as assistant co-ordinator to the project — something that Walter Barker supports as the next step in developing the programme.

Not 'cheap'

Walter Barker denies fiercely that it is a 'cheap option'; health authorities who see it as such are quickly put off when they realise there are on-costs after the initial outlay on training and materials, he claims. The Early childhood development unit charges some £16 000 over the first three years to train health visitors in first-

parent visiting, and a further £6000 for the community mothers programme. South East Kent, where a community mothers programme has just started, has allocated £20 000 to launch the scheme. The Nottingham budget is £30 000 a year basic, and extra 'inner-city funding' is being applied for.

Walter Barker is equally clear that the programme is not intended as a substitute for qualified health visitors. The aim is to complement the routine health visiting service.

'Health visitors are carrying the very considerable burden of crisis caseloads. They don't have the resources and the time to support every family.' Communities must be more involved 'at the grass roots' in their own health care.

'These women talk the same language as the families they visit, live in the same environment. Some of the community mothers themselves have experienced the kinds of problems faced by many of those they visit. Such experience gives them added credibility.

'I'm not saying health visitors haven't been in that position, but it's much less likely', he says.

Kate Billingham says that ideally Nottingham 'would employ more Asian health visitors — if we had them. But Asian babies have a high mortality rate and mothers are suffering. In terms of service provision, Asian women are getting a better service than they ever had before.'

She stresses, 'we need to recognise the knowledge and ability of women themselves.'.

The project 'is something we would have done whether we had a full health visiting establishment or not', says Celia Suppiah. 'It's not a way of propping up health visiting services. They are a voice for the health visitors to clients who perhaps aren't accepting the service. 'They encourage clients to make better use of health services. It's a way to cross the professional/client gap. It's involving the community in its own health care ■

Community mothers and health visitors from the Tilbury programme will be speaking at this year's HVA annual professional conference in October. Until then, they ask HVA members to understand that the programme is still in its early stages and they are not able to take individual enquiries but requests for further information can be made to locality manager: Ms Clare Trencher ☎ 0375 383676 x214.

CORONARY HEART DISEASE
AND STROKE

Example 2

Good practice pointers:

Meeting a need

- Started by identifying a need.

Involving the client

- Willingness to participate was important to the success of the project.

Defining the project clearly

- Clearly defined: objective/target; process of implementation; roles and responsibilities; evaluation plan; action plan and timetable.

Using healthy alliances

- Commitment extended beyond the health visitors to other professions.

Targeting the service

- Focused on families and used a multidisciplinary group to identify those at risk.

Choosing the right location

- Location chosen to meet client preferences. Costs and benefits of different locations assessed before choosing.

Seeking advice from others

- Evidence of success from elsewhere, and advice from the HVA and the HEA was used.

Improving diet for low-income families

A group of health visitors were particularly concerned about the inadequate diets of many young mothers and their children in areas with a high proportion of low income families. They were aware of larger than average numbers of children with low birth weights, failure to thrive, obesity, high levels of dental caries and referrals to speech therapy.

Inadequate diet was partly caused by a lack of formal education and parental role modelling, which led to the use of prepackaged instant meals. The health visitors knew that the parents were keen to do their best from the excellent response to nutrition displays in the area, such as a 'healthy eating' stall set up in the local market to demonstrate healthy packed school lunches. However, the parents lacked a basic knowledge of nutrition, shopping, meal planning, budgeting and cooking.

A multidisciplinary group of health visitor's, Health Promotion Officers and a Community Dietician planned the development of a practice targeted at specific families. They sought advice from the HVA and the Health Promotion Unit regarding the type of projects with a proven track record This group specified the teaching aims, the content of the programmes and the evaluation methods. Full documentation was prepared.

Other professionals involved at different stages include the School Nurse, Community Dental Officer and Speech Therapist.

'At risk' families were identified by professionals from different disciplines working in the community. The families were invited to participate in a series of sessions which were designed to improve nutrition.

The groups, of approximately 10 parents (with children) meet over six lunch times. The sessions are held in public venues such as local pubs, community centres and

Developing the service

- Service developed to meet new needs as they were identified.

Evaluating the service

- Formal evaluation is used - changed nutrition levels; eating habits of individual families; clients' perception of usefulness; the acceptability of style of provision, and clinical indicators such as weight loss/gain.

- Evaluation criteria adapted to meet changing circumstances.

- Initiative costed fully; cost utility evaluations are planned.

Spreading the word

- Many people have been informed; education and training has actively changed in response to this.

church halls and are facilitated by a health visitor. The session content varies according to the families' needs, but typically includes:

- preparing and sharing a meal

- discussions about shopping and best value choices

- introduction to healthy eating messages using the plate method and food group system

- nutritional labelling,

- prices, costs and comparisons

- budgeting for meals,

- planning meals

- preparing meals for families, children, parties

- healthy, cheap and easy foods.

Clients have started to ask for recipe books for the meals prepared. These are being adapted in a sensitive way as there is an above average rate of illiteracy amongst this group of parents.

Success is evaluated in a number of ways - by reference to a diet 'diary' completed before the groups begins, immediately after, and six months later. This is assessed by the community dietician. They also evaluate 'quality' through a client satisfaction survey.

Results already show changed dietary habits and improvement in nutritional intake of those participating. There is also an improvement in mothers' self esteem and willingness to change. This will soon become part of the formal evaluation of practice.

The health visitors hope that the members of the group will join in the planning, running and evaluation of the group as it develops. They also anticipate that some members may go on and help in other groups.

CORONARY HEART DISEASE
AND STROKE

Example 2 continued

The initiative has been costed fully, and there are plans to carry out cost utility evaluations when the data is available.

They will use the project as a resource for nurse students. There are four Community Practice Teachers within the community nursing team who conduct training on a regular basis. Health visitors, district nurses and P2000 students will be involved in this partnership. They have also written up the project in the Health Services Journal, and won the Health Visitors Association and National Dairy Council award of £5,000.

Contact

Debbie Stubberfield, Parkway Health Centre, Parkway, New Addington, Croydon, Surrey. Tel: 0689 842117.

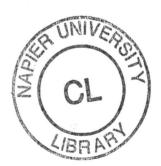

MENTAL ILLNESS

Example 1

> **Good practice pointers:**
>
> **Keeping on target**
>
> - Pre-dates "Health of the Nation" but is aimed at the general objective of improving the health and social functioning of mentally ill people.
>
> **Using healthy alliances**
>
> - Involves a multidisciplinary Health Authority/University team.
>
> **Researching the approach**
>
> - National and local epidemiological and other relevant data were reviewed.
>
> - Nurses, midwives and health visitors need to know the data on various treatment regimes and be clear about how this data affects their practice.
>
> **Improving access**
>
> - Accessibility to patients is improved through being available without appointment.
>
> - Speedy assessment policy help towards achieving "Health of the Nation" targets.
>
> **Documenting the process**
>
> - Comprehensive documentation is a key principle of good practice.

Providing post-natal day services

This initiative provides day hospital facilities for women suffering from psychological problems related to child birth. The service was introduced in a psychiatric day hospital in 1986. It has places for up to eight babies; the number of mothers treated depends upon access to nursery provision.

The initiative demonstrates a unique partnership between the North Staffordshire Health Authority and the Department of Post Graduate Medicine at the University of Keele. The service is provided by a multidisciplinary team of staff.

There is formal documentation showing the processes and procedures for assessment, admission, referral, treatment, prevention, discharge, support and so on. The documentation includes copies of the formal assessment and patient satisfaction survey forms used.

Staff have adopted the philosophy of holistic care. They use a variety of interventions because they believe that there is no single causal factor of post natal psychological disorders.

Preventing and caring

- Supporting those already diagnosed as having post natal depression and preventing its occurrence.

Evaluating the service

- Formal evaluation is planned to measure the reduction in suicides and the improved health and well-being of patients.

Spreading the word

- Disseminating practice to those who need to know.

The service has an open referral system including self referral/drop in patients. There is a two week maximum waiting time for an appointment/assessment.

The unit counsels parents whose personal or family history puts them at high risk of experiencing child bearing-related psychiatric disorders. Advice on pre-conception and post-natal counselling is given to mothers who have had previous puerperal psychosis.

The unit plans to encourage research into the effectiveness of its service. There is a formal patient satisfaction questionnaire.

They have taken considerable steps to make their service known to the local public and to staff in the district and region. Media used include national and local press and the TV. The team won a Hospital Doctor Psychiatric Team award in 1992.

Contact

Mrs Janice Gerrard (Unit Manager), Patient and Baby Day Unit, 17 Charles Street, Hanley, North Staffordshire, Tel: 0782 268945

And today's remedy will be ...

The Government is not short of new initiatives for NHS reform. But it seems to be making policy up as it goes along, and lacks a clear strategy for the future of the service, argues CHRIS HAM in today's British Medical Journal.

LAST WEEK a series of reports was published on the role of the Department of Health and the management of the new National Health Service. These reports were commissioned in the light of the functions and manpower review and the decision to abolish regional health authorities and merge district health authorities and family health services authorities. The result of ministerial deliberations and Treasury intervention will be a substantial reduction in the number of civil servants in the Department of Health. There will also be tight controls over the number of staff employed in the new regional offices of the NHS Executive and a move to accelerate joint commissioning between district health authorities and family health services authorities. This all adds up to a further period of major structural change as the Government seeks to get the organisation right.

While many of the planned changes are sensible in their own right, taken together they will undoubtedly divert scarce managerial time and attention away from the real issues facing the health services. These are less to do with structure and management than with the future direction of the NHS itself. As things stand, there is no coherent strategy guiding the development of the NHS, and there is a suspicion that the current occupants of Richmond House are not much interested in developing one. Tactics have come to dominate strategy, and ministers have seemed more concerned with keeping the NHS out of the headlines than with articulating a clear vision for the future.

Some people will argue that this is unfair and ignores the health strategy set out in The Health Of The Nation for England and in its sister documents for the rest of the United Kingdom. While this argument has some validity, it does not explain how The Health Of The Nation is to be reconciled with the very wide range of other policy initiatives to emerge from the Department of Health. To name but a few, the Patient's Charter, the policy on community care, the efficiency index and the reduction of junior doctor's hours have all, at different times, been given priority by the Government, suggesting a lack of clarity at the centre on what really matters. This is not new; but the proliferation of policies from the Department of Health has entered an acute phase, well illustrated by the NHS Executive's business plan for 1994/95 which includes no fewer than 83 objectives.

Matters are made worse by the inconsistency of current policies. Whereas the efficiency index requires health authorities to increased workload in the acute sector to satisfy the Treasury's demands, The Health Of The Nation and the development of community care call for a reallocation of resources away from hospitals. This sends out a signal that the left hand may not always be sure of what the right hand is doing. Faced with multiple and conflicting demands, NHS managers can be forgiven for feeling confused. At a time when many managers find themselves embattled by thinly-veiled attacks on men in grey suits, ministers are at risk of achieving the unlikely feat of uniting doctors and managers in a common cause against Government policies.

Even more significantly, there has been little debate about the direction in which health services will develop in the longer term. To be sure, Mrs Bottomley did venture a few thoughts on the future of hospitals in a recent conference speech, but this was more an exercise in kite flying than a carefully thought out analysis of the issues. The reality is that short-term political horizons dominate the thinking of politicians and militate against debate on matters of more fundamental importance. This has left a vacuum that civil servants, themselves preoccupied with organisational changes and steering the implementation of the NHS reforms, have shown no inclination to fill.

Underlying many of these issues is continuing uncertainty about the evolution of the NHS reforms. Unlike previous reorganisations, the changes introduced by Working For Patients were sketched in broad outline only, with many of the most important details missing. This reflected the tight timetable against which the White Paper was prepared and the fact that most of the central ideas in the reforms had been only partially thought through. There has, therefore, been no overall plan guiding the implementation of the reforms and little sense of where they will ultimately lead. In business-school parlance, Working For Patients is best described as an emergent strategy. Expressed in more simple language, ministers have been making it up as they have been going along. For many managers and professionals in the NHS, this has means a period of learning by doing, in which the importance of GP fund-holding, NHS trusts, and similar initiatives have been discovered in the process of making the reforms work. Where these changes will take the NHS is unclear even (or perhaps especially) to those at the heart of government.

Consequently, many of the most important questions about the reforms remain un-answered. These include the balance that will be struck between competition and management, the relation between fund-holding and health-authority commissioning and the number and configuration of NHS trusts. The reality is that the way in which these issues are resolved will depend as much on how the reforms develop locally as on ministers' decisions. To this extent, the changes introduced by Working For Patients are out of control, with developments being driven from the bottom up, not from the top down.

And yet despite the over-whelming evidence of confusion and inconsistency at the centre of the NHS, there are those who argue that the reforms are guided by a master plan, designed to destabilise established relationships and to undermine the very principles on which the NHS was established. This conspiracy theory holds that ministers are pursuing a hidden agenda which, through a series of incremental steps, will result in more private involvement in the financing and delivery of health services. The difficulty with this argument is that not only are politicians not that clever, but also that for any government to undermine the NHS, however surreptitiously, would be electoral suicide. In practice, health policy is more the result of cock-up than conspiracy, and the time has now come to address some of the ambiguities that exist.

What should be done? First, ministers should assess the founding principles of the NHS for their relevance today. This applies not only to the principles of access and equity, which have come under pressure as the NHS market has begun to bite, but also to the principles of comprehensiveness. The decision by the ombudsman that the NHS has an obligation to provide nursing care to patients who are seriously ill will intensify the debate about rationing. This issue can no longer be avoided, and ministers should immediately initiate a debate about the scope of the NHS, following the example of their counterparts in Sweden, the Netherlands, and New Zealand.

Alongside this debate, ministers should clarify where they see the current reforms taking the NHS in the longer term. This will not be possible in great detail, but at a minimum, there should be greater clarity about the principles of market management, the nature of the purchasing function and the development of NHS trusts. Four years into the implementation of the reforms there is sufficient experience to fill the gaps in Working For Patients and to spell out the direction of change in the next phase of development. This would enable the legitimate (as opposed to partisan) claims of the medical profession and other interests to be taken into account in a refinement of the reforms. In this respect, ministers should place the emphasis on contestability rather than competitive tendering of clinical services, build in stronger incentives for improved performance and address the growing problem of morale in general practice.

The other priority is to articulate a vision of the future of health services themselves. This includes taking into account the impact of technological advances and demographic changes and ensuring that services develop in line with research evidence on the most appropriate and effective location of medical care. This may entail the politically uncomfortable acceptance that market principles won't guarantee the concentration of services in centres that produce the best results. These issues need to be addressed alongside issues to do with structure and management.

Chris Ham is Director of the Health Services Management Centre, University of Birmingham

GENERAL PRACTICE

Effectiveness of health checks conducted by nurses in primary care: final results of the OXCHECK study

Imperial Cancer Research Fund OXCHECK Study Group

See pp 1105, 1109 and editorial by Toon

University of Oxford,
Department of Public
Health and Primary Care,
Gibson Building, Radcliffe
Infirmary, Oxford
OX2 6HE
Members of the OXCHECK
Study Group are:

University Department of
Public Health and Primary
Care
A Coulter, G Fowler,
A Fuller, L Jones,
T Lancaster, M Lawrence,
D Mant, J Muir, A Neil,
C O'Neil, L Roe, N Rusted,
T Schofield, C Silagy,
M Thorogood. P Yudkin,
S Ziebland

Chemical Pathology
Department, Luton and
Dunstable District General
Hospital
D Freedman, M Oggelsby,
S Joyce, Y Sweetman

Department of Biological
Sciences, Sheffield Hallam
University
R F Smith

Participating general
practitioners
P Bradley, R Brown,
S Choudhury, M Clarke,
J Crarer, D Denis-
Smith, H Francis,
P Maddock, J Marsden,
D Marshall, S Martin,
H McGill, A Mitchell,
O O'Toole, M Roberts,
C Royall, A Sander,
J Stanton, H Swallow,
C Sykes, J Tabert, S Talbot,
D Tant, M Waldron,
P Williams

Participating practice
nurses
I Allen, S Brown, P Clark,
J Draper, P Gazeley,
S Lilley. K Mustoe, J Steele,
J Szumski, M Tyrrell,
K Tiernan, J Vanderwall,
S Vella, A White, K Warren,
A White, P Wolsey,
L Young

Report prepared by J Muir.
T Lancaster, L Jones,
P Yudkin

Correspondence to:
Dr Muir.

BMJ 1995;310:1099-1104

Abstract

Objective—To determine the effectiveness of health checks, performed by nurses in primary care, in reducing risk factors for cardiovascular disease and cancer.

Design—Randomised controlled trial.

Setting—Five urban general practices in Bedfordshire.

Subjects—2205 men and women who were randomly allocated a first health check in 1989-90 and a re-examination in 1992-3 (the intervention group); 1916 men and women who were randomly allocated an initial health check in 1992-3 (the control group). All subjects were aged 35-64 at recruitment in 1989.

Main outcome measures—Serum total cholesterol concentration, blood pressure, body mass index, and smoking prevalence (with biochemical validation of cessation); self reported dietary, exercise, and alcohol habits.

Results—Mean serum total cholesterol was 3·1% lower in the intervention group than controls (difference 0·19 mmol/l (95% confidence interval 0·12 to 0·26)); in women it was 4·5% lower (P < 0·0001) and in men 1·6% (P < 0·05), a significant difference between the sexes (P < 0·01). Self reported saturated fat intake was also significantly lower in the intervention group. Systolic and diastolic blood pressures and body mass index were respectively 1·9%, 1·9%, and 1·4% lower in the intervention group (P < 0·005 in all cases). There was a 3·9% (2·4 to 5·3) difference in the percentage of subjects with a cholesterol concentration ≥8 mmol/l, but no significant differences in the number with diastolic blood pressure ≥100 mm Hg or body mass index ≥30 kg/m². There was no significant difference between the two groups in prevalence of smoking or excessive alcohol use. Annual rechecks were no more effective than a single recheck at three years, but health checks led to a significant increase in visits to the nurse according to patients' degree of cardiovascular risk.

Conclusions—The benefits of health checks were sustained over three years. The main effects were to promote dietary change and reduce cholesterol concentrations; small differences in blood pressure may have been attributable to accommodation to measurement. The benefits of systematic health promotion in primary care are real, but must be weighed against the costs in relation to other priorities.

Introduction

In 1994 we reported the effectiveness of general practice based, nurse run health checks after one year of follow up in the randomised controlled OXCHECK (Oxford and collaborators health check) trial. The main differences between the intervention and control groups were in serum total cholesterol concentration (2·3%), systolic blood pressure (2·5%), and diastolic blood pressure (2·4%). No significant differences in smoking prevalence or body mass index were detected. The Family Heart Study Group reported concurrently that a similar randomised intervention aimed at families led to a 16% difference at one year in the total coronary risk score (Dundee risk score[2]).[3]

These reports provoked extensive, and sometimes passionate, debate about the benefits and costs of systematic health promotion through primary care.[4-6] The 1990 contract offered general practitioners financial rewards for providing health checks, which were often performed by nurses. In 1992 the new health promotion package shifted the emphasis to opportunistic intervention, but it continued to encourage primary care teams to perform screening, record data on lifestyle, and offer intervention to their adult patients aged 16-74. Substantial resources are diverted from other areas of general practice to reward this activity, which is seen as central to achieving government targets for reducing heart disease and cancer incidence.[7] These public health benefits can be realised only if effects of primary care health promotion are sustained over time, but the extent to which this occurs is uncertain.[5] We addressed this issue.

Subjects and methods

The study was performed in five general practices in Luton and Dunstable. This area was chosen for its mixed urban and suburban setting, range of heavy and light industry, and varied demographic profile. It had the additional advantage that there was no facilitator in post encouraging practices to perform health checks. All five practices in Luton with over 10 000 patients were approached. Three agreed to take part, and two further practices, with lists of about 7500 were recruited, one of which was in Dunstable.

Potential participants were identified from the Bedfordshire Family Practitioner Committee's register in the autumn of 1988. The 17 965 men and women aged 35-64 who were identified were sent a health and lifestyle questionnaire. A total of 11 090 (80·3% after adjusting for inaccuracies of registration) returned the questionnaire, and they were randomly allocated in 1988 to health checks during one of the four years from 1989 to 1993. Invitation to health checks was by post, by telephone, and opportunistically during surgery visits. Considerable effort was invested to attain a target attendance rate of 80% of those who had been randomly allocated to each group.[1]

Our principal analysis is of the effects of the intervention after three years of follow up; figure 1 shows the groups compared. The intervention group consisted of the 2205 participants who attended their first health check in 1989-90 (year 1 of the study) and were scheduled for re-examination in 1992-3 (year 4 of the study). They were compared with 1916 controls who attended their first health check in 1992-3 (year 4).

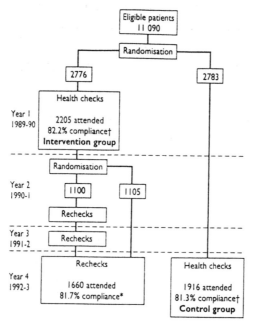

FIG 1—*Design of OXCHECK trial showing composition of intervention and control groups at three year follow up. A total of 5531 patients randomly allocated health checks in years 2 and 3 are excluded from this analysis*

* Denominator is all patients attending a first health check who were subsequently randomly allocated annual rechecks or a single recheck minus those who left the practice area before receiving the final recheck.

† Denominator is all patients randomly allocated to a first health check minus those who left the practice area before receiving it.

The 2205 participants allocated to a first health check in year 1 of the study were further randomly allocated annual re-examinations (1100) or a single return visit at three years (1105). We were thus able to examine the effect of annual rechecks. We also examined the effects of intervention in 2080 participants who had their first health check in the second year of the study, 1990-1, and were re-examined in 1992-3, two years after the intervention. The results in this group were consistent with those seen at three years, and the data are therefore not shown (available on request to JM).

Practice nurses performed health checks according to a standard protocol, which included completing a medical history, lifestyle questionnaire, and structured dietary assessment.[10] They measured height, weight (on Seca scales), and blood pressure (with the Hawksley random zero sphygmomanometer) and drew blood for determination of serum cholesterol concentration. Details of the laboratory methods have been previously reported.[1] Patients were offered follow up according to a structured protocol for each risk factor. Initial health checks took 45-60 minutes, and follow up visits 10-20 minutes. Nurses were instructed in the importance of identifying and following up patients with multiple risk factors and in the use of a patient centred communication model.[11] They attended a two day induction course, an annual study day, and a monthly evening training session with the medical and nursing coordinators to maintain and develop their knowledge and skills. In some practices nurses in post combined health checks with other work, while in others nurses were employed specifically to perform health checks. Over the course of the study each practice required roughly 50 hours a week of a nurse's time.

Results are presented both for those who attended for re-examination and for all patients scheduled to attend on the assumption that non-attenders showed no change from their initial visit or last recheck (analysis by intention to treat). This assumption is generally conservative, except in the case of cholesterol concentration and blood pressure, which rise with age. The effect of this assumption was modelled by adjusting the means for those with missing values at recheck for age related changes. The effects were

negligible (a 0·01 mmol/l difference in cholesterol concentration in women only), and unadjusted values were therefore used in subsequent analysis. Subjects classed as smokers at the initial health check were considered to be non-smokers at follow up only if their report of having given up smoking was confirmed by measurement of serum cotinine concentration.

The notes of 1100 patients in the intervention group with a raised blood pressure (≥160 mm Hg systolic or ≥90 mm Hg diastolic) or cholesterol concentration (≥8·0 mmol/l) identified at the health check were audited at the end of the study to determine how many patients were prescribed pharmaceutical treatment after the checks. In addition, the notes of 1000 consecutive patients attending for a health check were audited to ascertain the annual rates of consultation with doctors and nurses in the year before and after a first health check.

Confidence intervals were calculated with the confidence interval analysis program.[12] The means of continuous variables were compared between the two groups and the significance of differences was assessed by the t test. The χ^2 test was used to test the significance of differences in proportions. Minor inconsistencies in the tables reflect rounding or missing values for some variables. The study was approved by the Central Oxford Ethics Committee.

Results

As previously reported, the groups randomly allocated at baseline to a health check during each year of the trial did not differ significantly in the distribution of age or social class.

Table I shows the mean differences in total cholesterol concentration, blood pressure, and body mass index between the intervention and control groups for attenders at re-examination and for all patients scheduled to attend after three years of follow up. The true effect of health checks in this trial is likely to lie between the two estimates, but we present the intention to treat analysis as the principal outcome of the trial.

Cholesterol concentration, blood pressure, and body mass index differed significantly. Mean total cholesterol concentration was 3·1% lower in the intervention than in the control group (P<0·0001); in women it was 4·5% lower (P<0·0001) and in men 1·6% (P<0·05). This difference between the sexes was significant (difference 0·18 mmol/l (95% confidence interval 0·04 to 0·32), P<0·01). The mean systolic and diastolic blood pressures and body mass index were lower in the intervention group by 1·9% (P<0·0001), 1·9% (P<0·0001), and 1·4% (P<0·005) respectively. When the analysis was restricted to those who re-attended, the differences for systolic and diastolic blood pressure and body mass index were the same but the differences in mean cholesterol concentration increased to 4·0% (women 5·2%, men 2·6%).

Table II shows differences in the proportions of patients in five high risk groups: smokers, those who were overweight, those with raised diastolic blood pressure or total cholesterol concentration, and those who drank alcohol excessively. The main significant difference was in the proportion with a high cholesterol concentration. Although the prevalence of smoking was lower in those attending a recheck, there was no significant difference in the intention to treat analysis. Figure 2 shows the frequency distribution of cholesterol concentrations in the intervention and control groups at three years. The curve for the intervention group lies to the left of that for the controls, indicating benefit from intervention at all serum cholesterol concentrations, though with greater effect at the upper end of the distribution.

TABLE I—*Total cholesterol concentrations, blood pressures, and body mass indices in control group and after three years of intervention. Values are means (SD)*

	Control group	Intervention group		Difference from control (95% confidence interval)	
		Attenders only	All participants	Attenders only	All participants*
		Men and women			
No of participants	1916	1660	2205		
Total cholesterol (mmol/l)	6·18 (1·17)	5·93 (1·06)	5·99 (1·10)	0·25 (0·18 to 0·33)	0·19 (0·12 to 0·26)
Blood pressure (mm Hg):					
Systolic	129·0 (20·4)	126·8 (19·6)	126·5 (19·3)	2·2 (0·9 to 3·5)	2·5 (1·3 to 3·7)
Diastolic	77·2 (11·7)	75·7 (11·5)	75·7 (11·6)	1·5 (0·7 to 2·3)	1·5 (0·8 to 2·2)
Body mass index (kg/m²)	26·26 (4·31)	25·89 (4·14)	25·88 (4·21)	0·37 (0·09 to 0·65)	0·38 (0·12 to 0·64)
		Men			
No of participants	885	738	987		
Total cholesterol (mmol/l)	6·09 (1·07)	5·93 (1·02)	5·99 (1·06)	0·16 (0·06 to 0·26)	0·10 (0·00 to 0·20)
Blood pressure (mm Hg):					
Systolic	131·2 (20·2)	128·8 (19·0)	128·7 (18·3)	2·4 (0·5 to 4·3)	2·5 (0·7 to 4·3)
Diastolic	78·6 (11·9)	77·1 (11·5)	77·4 (11·5)	1·5 (0·4 to 2·7)	1·2 (0·1 to 2·3)
Body mass index (kg/m²)	26·33 (3·50)	25·88 (3·39)	25·89 (3·44)	0·45 (0·11 to 0·79)	0·45 (0·12 to 0·76)
		Women			
No of participants	1031	922	1218		
Total cholesterol (mmol/l)	6·26 (1·25)	5·93 (1·10)	5·98 (1·13)	0·33 (0·22 to 0·44)	0·28 (0·18 to 0·38)
Blood pressure (mm Hg):					
Systolic	127·0 (20·5)	125·3 (20·0)	124·7 (19·9)	1·7 (−0·1 to 3·5)	2·3 (0·6 to 4·0)
Diastolic	76·0 (11·4)	74·6 (11·3)	74·3 (11·5)	1·4 (0·4 to 2·4)	1·7 (0·7 tp 2·7)
Body mass index (kg/m²)	26·20 (4·90)	25·90 (4·65)	25·86 (4·74)	0·30 (−0·13 to 0·73)	0·34 (−0·06 to 0·74)

*Last value from health check or recheck for non-attenders.

TABLE II—*Numbers (percentages) of patients in high risk categories in control group and after three years of intervention*

	Control group	Intervention group		Difference from control (95% confidence interval)	
		Attenders only	All participants	Attenders only	All participants*
		Men and women			
No of participants	1916	1660	2205		
Smoking†	506 (26·4)	356 (21·4)	552 (25·0)	5·0 (2·2 to 7·8)	1·4 (−1·3 to 4·1)
Alcohol use‡	210 (11·0)	156 (9·4)	229 (10·4)	1·6 (−0·42 to 0·04)	0·6 (−1·3 to 2·5)
Total cholesterol ≥8 mmol/l	148 (7·8)	49 (3·1)	82 (3·9)	4·7 (3·2 to 6·2)	3·9 (2·4 to 5·3)
Diastolic pressure ≥100 mm Hg	86 (4·5)	53 (3·3)	73 (3·4)	1·2 (−0·1 to 2·5)	1·1 (−0·1 to 2·3)
Body mass index ≥30 kg/m²	304 (15·9)	220 (13·5)	310 (14·3)	2·4 (0·0 to 4·7)	1·6 (−0·6 to 3·8)
		Men			
No of participants	885	738	987		
Smoking†	270 (30·5)	190 (25·7)	296 (30·0)	4·8 (0·4 to 9·1)	0·5 (−3·7 to 4·7)
Alcohol use‡	155 (17·5)	112 (15·2)	164 (16·6)	2·3 (−1·3 to 5·9)	0·9 (−2·5 to 4·3)
Total cholesterol ≥8 mmol/l	56 (6·4)	19 (2·7)	34 (3·6)	3·7 (1·7 to 5·7)	2·8 (0·8 to 4·8)
Diastolic pressure ≥100 mm Hg	49 (5·5)	28 (3·9)	39 (4·0)	1·6 (−0·4 to 3·7)	1·5 (−0·4 to 3·5)
Body mass index ≥30 kg/m²	114 (12·9)	73 (10·1)	103 (10·6)	2·8 (−0·3 to 5·9)	2·3 (−0·6 to 5·2)
		Women			
No of participants	1031	922	1218		
Smoking†	236 (22·9)	166 (18·0)	256 (21·0)	4·9 (1·3 to 8·5)	1·9 (−1·6 to 5·3)
Alcohol use‡	55 (5·3)	44 (4·8)	65 (5·3)	0·6 (−1·4 to 2·5)	0·0 (−1·9 to 1·9)
Total cholesterol ≥8 mmol/l	92 (9·0)	30 (3·4)	48 (4·1)	5·6 (3·4 to 7·7)	4·8 (2·7 to 6·9)
Diastolic pressure ≥100 mm Hg	37 (3·6)	25 (2·8)	34 (2·9)	0·8 (−0·8 to 2·4)	0·7 (−0·7 to 2·2)
Body mass index ≥30 kg/m²	190 (18·4)	147 (16·3)	207 (17·3)	2·2 (−1·2 to 5·6)	1·2 (−2·0 to 4·4)

*Last value from health check or recheck used for non-attenders.
†Smoking any form of tobacco at least daily.
‡Reported weekly intake of >21 units for men and >14 units for women.

The prescribing audit showed that 28 out of 90 (30%) participants with a cholesterol concentration ≥8 mmol/l at the first health check were prescribed cholesterol lowering drugs. Of 215 patients with either a systolic blood pressure ≥160 mm Hg or a diastolic ≥90 mm Hg, 48 (22%) had been taking hypotensive drugs and 23 (11%) received such treatment after the health checks.

Table III shows the differences between intervention and control groups in reported diet and exercise. The proportion of patients reporting taking vigorous exercise less than once a month was significantly lower in the intervention group (difference 3·3% (0·5 to 6·1)). After intervention there was a 8·7% (6·0 to 11·4) difference in the proportions who used mainly butter or hard margarine and a 7·5% (4·8 to 10·3) difference in the proportion who drank mainly full cream milk.

We further examined the 2205 subjects who received their first health check in year 1 and compared the values at the final health check between 1100 randomly allocated to return for annual rechecks and 1105 randomly allocated to return for a recheck only at

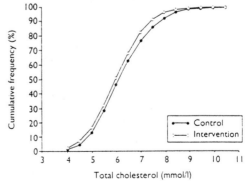

FIG 2—*Cumulative frequency distributions of total cholesterol concentration in control and intervention groups.*

three years. Values in the two groups were similar. Mean differences were: cholesterol −0·03 (−0·12 to 0·06) mmol/l, systolic blood pressure 0·2 (−1·4 to 1·8) mm Hg, diastolic blood pressure 0·0 (−1·0 to 1·0) mm Hg, and body mass index 0·29 (−0·06 to 0·64) kg/m². The difference in the proportion smoking was 1% (−2·6% to 4·6%).

TABLE III—*Reported diet and exercise in control group and after three years of intervention. Values are numbers (percentages) of patients unless stated otherwise*

	Control group	Intervention group		Difference from control (95% confidence interval)	
		Attenders only	All participants	Attenders only	All participants
Men and women					
No of participants	1916	1660	2205		
Exercise < once per month	1354 (70·9)	1094 (66·5)	1478 (67·6)	4·5 (1·4 to 7·5)	3·3 (0·5 to 6·1)
Use full cream milk	587 (30·6)	300 (18·5)	501 (23·1)	12·1 (9·4 to 15·0)	7·5 (4·8 to 10·3)
Use butter or hard margarine	587 (30·7)	303 (18·3)	483 (21·9)	12·4 (9·6 to 15·2)	8·7 (6·0 to 11·4)
Men					
No of participants	885	738	987		
Exercise < once per month	635 (71·8)	479 (65·4)	648 (66·2)	6·4 (1·9 to 10·9)	5·6 (1·5 to 9·8)
Use full cream milk	312 (35·3)	162 (22·4)	260 (26·7)	12·8 (8·5 to 17·2)	8·5 (4·3 to 12·7)
Use butter or hard margarine	286 (32·3)	141 (19·1)	232 (23·5)	13·2 (9·0 to 17·4)	8·8 (4·8 to 12·9)
Women					
No of participants	1031	922	1218		
Exercise < once per month	719 (70·1)	615 (67·3)	830 (68·8)	2·9 (−1·3 to 7·0)	1·4 (−2·5 to 5·2)
Use full cream milk	275 (26·7)	138 (15·3)	241 (20·1)	11·4 (7·8 to 15·0)	6·6 (3·1 to 10·1)
Use butter or hard margarine	301 (29·2)	162 (17·6)	251 (20·7)	11·6 (7·9 to 15·3)	8·6 (5·0 to 12·2)

Audit of the notes of 1000 patients attending for a health check showed that visits to the general practitioner did not increase in the year after an initial health check, but there were significant increases in visits to the nurse. In the first year after the health check, patients with none of four identified risk factors (raised cholesterol concentration, raised blood pressure, obesity, and smoking) had a mean number of 0·6 (0·4 to 0·8) visits to the nurse. For patients with one, two, and three or more risk factors the figures were respectively 1·3 (1·2 to 1·4), 1·6 (1·4 to 1·8), and 2·5 (2·1 to 2·9). In contrast, the mean number of visits in the year before the first health check was 0·3 (0·2 to 0·4) and did not differ according to number of risk factors. Women were twice as likely to visit the nurse as were men.

Discussion

To assess the effects over time of an intervention which included both screening and treatment presented several methodological problems. To collect data on a control group at baseline risked obscuring the benefits of health checks because of the similarity between measurement and intervention. We therefore randomly allocated patients to a health check in one of four successive years. This allowed us to compare those returning for rechecks after three years with a control group attending at the same time for their first health check, the control group thus having a low probability of contamination by previous contact with the study. The main concern with this design was the potential bias introduced by non-attendance for follow up in the intervention group. By analysing on intention to treat, we made a generally conservative assumption about the direction of this bias. Some of the non-attenders may, however, have changed their behaviours as a result of the health checks, particularly when the reason for non-attendance was because of having moved out of the area. Thus, our analysis may underestimate the impact of the health checks.

Any programme subjected to evaluation in general practice should be of high quality and generalisable. The nurses who provided the intervention were trained in the identification and modification of risk factors and in the use of a communication model that emphasised the importance of identifying and responding to the patients' concerns about their health, negotiating change according to patients' priorities, and reinforcing change through supportive follow up. Analysis of over 100 audiotapes of the checks with the nurses in this study met these standards in a high proportion of cases (T Schofield, personal communication). Our audit of subsequent visits showed that nurses were also

effective in stratifying risk and adjusting the intensity of follow up accordingly. Our reported results should therefore be seen in the context of high quality clinical performance by the nurses.

SMOKING

The lack of effectiveness of health checks in promoting stopping smoking confirms the disappointing findings from our one year follow up.[1] Perhaps this is not surprising. Studies showing an increase in stopping smoking after brief advice in primary care were performed over a decade ago.[13 14] As the prevalence of smoking has fallen, the proportion of smokers who can relinquish the habit with information and support alone has almost certainly fallen. Pharmacological treatments of proved efficacy now exist to supplement approaches based on behavioural and counselling models.[15] Making effective use of this array of methods for treating addictive behaviour may not be compatible with achieving the multiple tasks of a general health check.

BLOOD PRESSURE

The significant differences in mean blood pressures between the intervention and control groups are difficult to interpret because the size of the change is compatible with accommodation to measurement (the tendency of blood pressure recordings to yield lower values over time as subjects become used to the procedure).[16] Change in mean blood pressure may be due to screening and drug treatment of previously unidentified or inadequately treated hypertension or to the effects of advice on lifestyle in patients with the full range of blood pressure. The prevalence of moderate to severe hypertension at first attendance was low: only 4·5% of patients in the intervention group had a diastolic blood pressure greater than 100 mm Hg. This may be partly explained by underestimation of blood pressure by the Hawksley random zero sphygmomanometer.[17] It also suggests, however, that when opportunistic screening is already occurring, the yield of patients with undiagnosed or inadequately treated hypertension from systematic screening may be relatively low. The effects on population mean blood pressure of advice on lifestyle offered through a health check seem to be small at best.

DIET, CHOLESTEROL CONCENTRATION, AND WEIGHT

The most encouraging aspect of this trial was the evidence that dietary advice from nurses led to significant differences in self reported dietary and exercise habits and to a modest difference in the mean cholesterol concentrations. These effects were significant in both men and women and were sustained three years after the initial intervention. The frequency distribution curves of cholesterol concentration in figure 2 suggest that health checks had an effect on the diet of many subjects with average cholesterol concentration, in whom the attributable risk of ischaemic heart disease due to cholesterol is highest. That the effects on cholesterol concentration largely reflect dietary change is supported both by the differences in self reported saturated fat intake and by the small number of prescriptions for lipid lowering drugs. Dietary advice also led to a small difference in mean body mass index but failed to reduce the proportion of the population with obesity.

The magnitude of the effect on cholesterol concentration is comparable with the reductions of up to 4·0% reported in an overview of five trials of individualised advice on a reduced fat diet.[18] It is also consistent with our recently completed randomised trial of dietary advice in patients with raised cholesterol concentration (6·0-8·5 mmol/l), which found a mean difference in total cholesterol concentration of 1·5% at six months, after correction for regression to the mean.[19] The benefits of dietary advice are probably not fully reflected by measurements of cholesterol concentration. Reducing fat intake and substituting fruit and vegetables may raise serum concentrations of antioxidant vitamins and other cardioprotective factors, depite having little effect on lipid values.[19] Substantial epidemiological evidence suggests that this could reduce the risk of cancer and cardiovascular disease.[20] Such benefits must, however, remain speculative in the absence of data from clinical trials.

There may be several reasons why the intervention was more successful in changing diet than in effecting other behavioural changes. Modifying the diet, particularly when palatable substitutes exist for foodstuffs high in saturated fat, is probably an easier task than losing weight, curbing alcohol use, or breaking an addiction to smoking. In addition, the effect of advice may have been to validate information about healthy eating received from other sources. Whereas most smokers are aware of the harmful nature of their addiction,[21] confusion about public health messages on nutrition is well documented.[21 22] Advice from nurses may have catalysed changes previously contemplated.[23] Finally, the nurses may have invested greater effort in diet than in other issues as a result of the emphasis on collection of detailed dietary data in the health check protocol. It is unclear whether this represents the most efficient method of delivering dietary advice. Indeed, in another, shorter, randomised trial in general practice dietary advice was no more effective than written information in lowering cholesterol concentration.[19]

EFFECT OF ANNUAL RECHECKS

There was no evidence that annual rechecks after an initial health check were any more effective in modifying risk factors after three years than a single health check. The narrow confidence intervals around the differences between the two groups suggest that no important incremental effect was undetected. Our audit of clinical records shows, however, that health checks generated a significant number of follow up visits in both groups—up to four times more in patients with three or more risk factors. It would therefore be misleading to suggest that all the benefit of intervention can be realised by a single health check.

PUBLIC HEALTH BENEFITS

Caution is required in estimating effects on morbidity and mortality from change in risk factors. It is, however, important to make a judgment about the benefits that might accrue if this programme were widely implemented. Little or no reduction in cancer incidence can be expected from systematic health checks because of their lack of effect on the prevalence of smoking and excessive alcohol use. To calculate the change in incidence of ischaemic heart disease that might result from their application, we used overviews of the effects of reducing cholesterol concentration and blood pressure that correct for the regression dilution bias.[24 25] The long term risk reduction in (combined fatal and non-fatal) myocardial infarction attributable to cholesterol reduction was projected to be 6% in men and 13% in women. The mean difference of 1·5 mm Hg in diastolic blood pressure, if not discounted as an accommodation effect, would add a further 7% reduction in long term risk of myocardial infarction and should also lead to fewer strokes. These estimates are comparable with the overall 12% reduction in risk of myocardial infarction predicted by the Family Heart Study Group on the basis of its one year results.[1] In a population such effects might well be considered worth while. It is, however, important to understand the limitations of such projections, particularly among women, in whom the strength of the association between cholesterol concentration and cardiovascular risk remains contentious.[26]

The benefits of health checks will, moreover, only come to those who attend them. In this trial, subjects were recruited after they had expressed some interest in their health by completing an initial survey questionnaire.[1] Despite this, almost half of nurses' time in the OXCHECK trial was taken up with recruiting patients to health checks. A third of attenders at first health checks had required more than one invitation and a fifth failed to take up the offer even after three invitations. A third of those scheduled for follow up appointments failed to attend them. At best, two thirds of the target population received a health check, and about half attended for both an initial check and the agreed follow up. The effectiveness of the intervention was further attenuated by the poorer attendance rates of those at higher risk.[9] Moreover men, who face a higher absolute risk of cardiovascular disease, showed less change than the women, perhaps because they attended for follow up less frequently. Clearly, health checks cannot be seen as any more than one part of a population strategy for reducing cardiovascular disease.

CONCLUSIONS

The effects of health checks, especially on diet, were sustained after three years. A particular strength of our study is its generalisability. The intervention was provided in a representative general practice setting by nurses who received training that could realistically be offered nationally. Substantial resources were, however, devoted not only to this training but to recruitment, intervention, and follow up. We did not measure the psychological impact of health checks, but there is enough evidence from previous studies to be concerned that they are not without harm to individual patients.[27] The question is therefore not whether health checks work but whether they work enough to justify their costs. Formal cost effectiveness analysis of our data is in progress, but primary health care teams are already well aware of the opportunity costs of systematic health promotion. Few will wish to relinquish all responsibility for prevention in the light of our results. Many, however, may now share the view of Stott et al that, "Rewarding general practitioners for population coverage rather than using more sensitive and practical approaches to individuals is unlikely to build on the natural advantages of primary care."[7]

One final lesson from the OXCHECK trial is the difficulty of performing rigorous health services research to inform policy. The study began before

---

Key messages

- This study shows that health checks by nurses in primary care lead to sustained changes in dietary behaviour and a reduction of about 3% in serum cholesterol concentration; effects on blood pressure are of questionable significance

- There is little effect on smoking or alcohol use, and more targeted approaches to modifying these behaviours may be appropriate

- Systematic implementation of health checks might lead to a reduction in risk of myocardial infarction among those who attend of about 5-15%; men, who are at higher risk, show less change than women

- Health checks consume substantial resources, and their effect is attenuated by non-attendance

- The benefits of health promotion through primary care must be weighed against their costs and in relation to other priorities

---

offering health checks became part of general practitioners' contractual obligation in 1990. Before the first year results of the trial had been published, this policy had been abandoned and replaced by a strategy whose value was no more certain. If policy makers cannot wait for research it is crucial that they are ready to modify their programmes when evidence becomes available.

The study was funded by the Imperial Cancer Research Fund with additional funding from Upjohn and Parke-Davis. We thank Mr R Smith of Bedfordshire Family Health Services Authority for his sustained support of the study.

1 Imperial Cancer Research Fund OXCHECK Study Group. Effectiveness of health checks conducted by nurses in primary care: results of the OXCHECK study after one year. BMJ 1994;308:308-12.
2 Tunstall-Pedoe H. The Dundee coronary risk-disk for management of change in risk factors. BMJ 1991;303:744-7.
3 Family Heart Study Group. Randomised controlled trial evaluating cardio-vascular screening and intervention in general practice: principal results of British family heart study. BMJ 1994;308:313-20.
4 Mant D. Health checks—time to check out? Br J Gen Pract 1994;44:51-2.
5 Stott N. Screening for risk in general practice. BMJ 1994;308:285-6.
6 McCormick J. Health promotion: the ethical dimension. Lancet 1994;344: 390-1.
7 Secretary of State for Health. The health of the nation: a strategy for health in England. London: HMSO, 1992. (Cm 1986.)
8 Imperial Cancer Research Fund OXCHECK Study Group. Prevalence of risk factors for heart disease in OXCHECK trial: implications for screening in primary care. BMJ 1991;302:1057-60.
9 Thorogood M, Coulter A, Jones L, Yudkin P, Muir J, Mant D. Factors affecting response to an invitation to attend for a health check. J Epidemiol Community Health 1993;47:224-8.
10 Roe L, Strong C, Whiteside C, Neil A, Mant D. Dietary intervention in primary care: validity of the DINE method for diet assessment. Fam Pract 1994;11:375-81.
11 Schofield T. Communication. In: Fowler G, Gray M, Anderson P, eds. Prevention in general practice. Oxford: Oxford University Press, 1993:60-7.
12 Gardner SB, Winter PD, Gardner MJ. Confidence interval analysis (CIA). London: BMJ Publishing Group, 1991.
13 Jamrozik K, Vessey M, Fowler G, Wald N, Parker G, Vunakis HV. Controlled trial of three different anti smoking interventions in general practice. BMJ 1984;288:1449-503.
14 Russell MH, Wilson C, Taylor C, Baker CD. Effect of general practitioners' advice against smoking. BMJ 1979;ii:231-5.
15 Silagy C, Mant D, Fowler G, Lodge M. Meta-analysis on efficacy of nicotine replacement therapies in smoking cessation. Lancet 1994;343:139-42.
16 Medical Research Council Working Party. MRC trial of treatment of mild hypertension: principal results. BMJ 1985;291:97-104.
17 Conroy RM, O'Brien E, O'Malley K, Atkins N. Measurement error in the Hawksley random zero sphygmomanometer: what damage has been done and what can we learn? BMJ 1993;306:1319-22.
18 Ramsay LE, Yeo WW, Jackson PR. Dietary reduction of serum cholesterol concentration: time to think again. BMJ 1991;303:953-7.
19 Neil HAW, Roe L, Godlee RJP, Moore J, Clark GMG, Brown J, et al. Randomised trial of lipid lowering dietary advice in general practice: the effects on serum lipids, lipoproteins, and antioxidants. BMJ 1995;310: 469-73.
20 Manson JE, Gaziano JM, Jonas MA, Hennekens CH. Antioxidants and cardiovascular disease: a review. J Am Coll Nutr 1993;12:426-32.
21 Silagy C, Muir J, Coulter A, Thorogood M, Roe L. Cardiovascular risk and attitudes to lifestyle: what do patients think? BMJ 1993;306:1657-60.
22 Frankel S, Davison C, Smith GD. Lay epidemiology and the rationality of responses to health education. Br J Gen Pract 1991;41:428-30.
23 Prochaska JO, DiClemente CD. Stages and processes of self-change of smoking: toward an integrative model of change. J Consult Clin Psychol 1983;51:390-5.
24 Law MR, Wald NJ, Thompson SG. By how much and how quickly does reduction in serum cholesterol concentration lower risk of ischaemic heart disease? BMJ 1994;308:367-72.
25 Collins R, Peto R, MacMahon S, Hebert P, Fiebach NH, Eberlein KA, et al. Blood pressure, stroke, and coronary heart disease. II. Short-term reductions in blood pressure: overview of randomised drug trials in their epidemiological context. Lancet 1990;335:827-38.
26 Hulley SB, Walsh JMB, Newman TB. Health policy on blood cholesterol. Time to change direction. Circulation 1992;86:1026-9.
27 Haynes BR, Sackett DL, Taylor DW, Gibson ES, Johnson A. Increased absenteeism from work after detection and labelling of hypertensive patients. N Engl J Med 1978;299:741-4.
28 Stott NCH, Kinnersley P, Rollnick S. The limits to health promotion. BMJ 1994;309:971-2.

(Accepted 3 February 1995)

A MEMORABLE PATIENT

An African woman weeps

Theresa was waiting for an operation in an African hospital. But as there were so many patients her operation would have to be postponed for another day, or week, or perhaps months. Such postponements are common and the patients quietly wrap their covering sheets around themselves, pick up their medical records, and make their way back to the wards from the waiting area of the operating theatre. Disappointed as most patients are when this happens they are usually hopeful because to have got this far means that they will ultimately get their operation. But Theresa had lost hope and cried in a way that I had never seen an African woman cry before. As I passed I could see the tears just roll down her cheeks as she sat quietly and waited resigned and dignified. During my several working trips to Africa I had seen and heard many women cry in Africa. When the children die the mothers weep and wail and throw themselves on the floor in a way that is very disturbing but Theresa's tears were of a different kind and I was perplexed and curious.

From her medical history I could work out a large part of her story. She was probably from a remote part of Africa. Married at a young age her pregnancy and labour would have been poorly managed. Many hours of obstructed labour occurred before some form of delivery, most likely of a dead baby, was carried out. By that time the pressure of the baby's head on the mother's pelvis had damaged her bladder so badly that now she leaked urine continuously. Her vesicovaginal fistula needed major surgery. In some ways she was fortunate. She had not died in obstructed labour as so many thousands of women do in Africa. Eventually she had managed, no doubt with many difficulties, to find the means to travel perhaps over 50 km to our hospital where she was now waiting for some chance of a cure.

I called one of the nurses over to translate for me and to find some explanation for her weeping. It seemed that Theresa knew that the next day there was to be a government plan to start charging fees for operations. She was a poor woman without money. She thought that as her operation was to be postponed she had lost hope of a cure. All her previous waiting would be in vain and hence the tears.

Under pressure from the International Monetary Fund and the World Bank many powerless African governments have been forced to introduce cuts in health care and education and charge for treatment. Theresa's tears were the human consequences of these policies. No doubt there are many thousands of people like Theresa in Africa. The poorest of the poor are bearing a burden with their lives for the policies of the banks. The debt repayments, the arms trade, and the international unjust trade policies rob Africa of any economic progress. A new brutal and insidious slavery is being perpetuated.—RAY TOWEY is a consultant anaesthetist in London

Reprinted from the BRITISH MEDICAL JOURNAL, 29th January 1994, Vol. 308, Pages 313-320

Randomised controlled trial evaluating cardiovascular screening and intervention in general practice: principal results of British family heart study

Family Heart Study Group

The members of the Family Heart Study Group are:

Preventive Cardiology, Medicine, University of Southampton and Clinical Epidemiology, National Heart and Lung Institute, University of London
D A Wood

Primary Medical Care and Preventive Cardiology, Medicine, University of Southampton
A L Kinmonth, G A Davies, J Yarwood

Medical Statistics Unit, London School of Hygiene and Tropical Medicine
S G Thompson, S D M Pyke, Y Kok

Wolfson Research Laboratories, University of Birmingham
R Cramb, C Le Guen

Wellcome Psychology and Genetics Research Group, United Medical and Dental Schools of Guy's and St Thomas's Hospitals
T M Marteau

Department of Medicine, University of Manchester
P N Durrington

Report prepared by D A Wood, A-L Kinmonth, S D M Pyke, S G Thompson

Correspondence to:
Professor D A Wood, Department of Clinical Epidemiology, National Heart and Lung Institute, London SW3 6LY.

BMJ 1994;308:313-20

Abstract

Objective—To measure the change in cardiovascular risk factors achievable in families over one year by a cardiovascular screening and lifestyle intervention in general practice.

Design—Randomised controlled trial in 26 general practices in 13 towns in Britain.

Subjects—12 472 men aged 40-59 and their partners (7460 men and 5012 women) identified by household.

Intervention—Nurse led programme using a family centred approach with follow up according to degree of risk.

Main outcome measures—After one year the pairs of practices were compared for differences in (a) total coronary (Dundee) risk score and (b) cigarette smoking, weight, blood pressure, and random blood cholesterol and glucose concentrations.

Results—In men the overall reduction in coronary risk score was 16% (95% confidence interval 11% to 21%) in the intervention practices at one year. This was partitioned between systolic pressure (7%), smoking (5%), and cholesterol concentration (4%). The reduction for women was similar. For both sexes reported cigarette smoking at one year was lower by about 4%, systolic pressure by 7 mm Hg, diastolic pressure by 3 mm Hg, weight by 1 kg, and cholesterol concentration by 0·1 mmol/l, but there was no shift in glucose concentration. Weight, blood pressure, and cholesterol concentration showed the greatest difference at the top of the distribution. If maintained long term the differences in risk factors achieved would mean only a 12% reduction in risk of coronary events.

Conclusions—As most general practices are not using such an intensive programme the changes in coronary risk factors achieved by the voluntary health promotion package for primary care are likely to be even smaller. The government's screening policy cannot be justified by these results.

Introduction

The prevention of coronary heart disease and stroke is a priority for the government in the *Health of the Nation*.[1] Targets have been set for the major cardiovascular risk factors—smoking, diet in relation to obesity, and blood pressure—and a voluntary health promotion package for primary care aimed at modifying these factors, among both high risk groups and the population as a whole, is now being put in place.[2] Though practice teams can ascertain cardiovascular risk factors in their population,[3] the important question is whether intervention will result in a reduction in these risk factors.

The only randomised controlled trial of multifactorial screening reported from general practice showed no significant changes in morbidity or mortality during a nine year follow up of those screened compared with those offered conventional medical care.[4] Controlled trials of unifactorial interventions are scarce in general practice and restricted to smoking, blood pressure,

and diabetes. Trials of smoking cessation among unselected cigarette smokers in general practice have consistently reported a higher rate of stopping in the intervention group,[5] particularly for an intensive programme led by general practitioners.[6] More recently nicotine patches in motivated heavy cigarette smokers have proved to be an effective aid to stopping smoking.[7][8] The Medical Research Council's mild to moderate hypertension trial showed a significant reduction in the incidence of stroke, although not coronary heart disease, in those taking antihypertensive drugs[9]; but retrospective reviews of general practice records to assess the detection and management of hypertension have shown that patients who have their blood pressure measured are not necessarily investigated, followed up, and treated.[10-12] In a randomised comparison of care of patients with non-insulin dependent diabetes in hospital and general practice the group being cared for by their general practitioner had less regular follow up and higher glycated haemoglobin concentrations than those who attended hospital clinics.[13] So although intensive smoking interventions may lead to reduced cigarette consumption, little or no evidence from intervention studies supports the efficacy of the government's current health promotion package for primary care based on multifactorial risk factor assessment and lifestyle intervention.

The British family heart study addressed this issue in a randomised controlled trial of nurse led screening for cardiovascular risk factors and lifestyle intervention in families in general practices in towns throughout Britain.[14] The overall aim of the trial was to estimate the size of the change in cardiovascular risk factors in men and women that could be achieved by such a practice based strategy in one year. Specifically, the main objectives were to measure the effect of one year's intervention on (a) total coronary risk score assessed with the Dundee risk score[15] for three modifiable risk factors (cigarette smoking, blood pressure, and cholesterol concentration) and (b) the prevalence of cigarette smoking and the distribution of weight, blood pressure, and random blood cholesterol and glucose concentrations in the population.

Subjects and methods

DESIGN

The study design has already been described[14] and is summarised in figure 1. Fifteen towns were selected which met specific demographic criteria. Within each town all general practices with 4-7 full time partners were surveyed and a pair of willing practices in each town with similar sociodemographic characteristics was randomised to either arm of the study. Such a pair was successfully identified in 14 towns and the two practices in each town were then randomly allocated to either intervention or external comparison groups.

Research nurses were recruited locally and trained centrally in the Department of Clinical Epidemiology at the National Heart and Lung Institute, London. Training comprised questionnaire interviews on a lap top computer, measurement of risk factors, quality

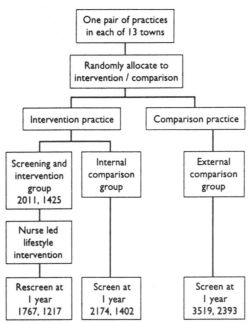

FIG 1—*Design of British family heart study showing numbers of men (first) and women seen at baseline and one year in the intervention group and at one year in the internal and external comparison groups*

assurance and follow up, and client centred counselling about lifestyle within families.

Identification of families suitable for recruitment to the study was by household through the male partner. The entire list of men aged 40-59 in each of the intervention and comparison practices was randomly ordered within five year age bands. In intervention practices each five year age band was randomly divided into two equal size groups: an intervention and internal comparison group. In the intervention group men and their families were approached in order (and at the same rate within each five year age band) by the nurses. Families were screened, offered risk related lifestyle intervention and follow up, and then rescreened after one year. Families in the internal or external comparison groups, although identified at the same time as those in the intervention groups, were first screened at one year at the same time as the intervention group was being rescreened.

SCREENING

Appointments were made by the nurses for each man and his family by telephoning the household. All family members attending were screened but only men and their partners were followed up. The initial screening interview for an adult couple in the intervention group lasted on average one and a half hours and for comparison families about half this time, the lifestyle intervention being less intensive. During the interview demographic, lifestyle, and medical information was recorded on computer and the following measurements were made: height and weight (Seca digital model 707 with telescopic measuring rod), body mass index (weight/height^2), carbon monoxide concentration in breath (Smokerlyzer), blood pressure (Takeda UA731 automatic digital sphygmomanometer), and random blood concentration of total cholesterol and glucose in a finger prick sample (Reflotron, Boehringer Mannheim); quality assurance was organised by the Wolfson Research Laboratories, Birmingham. In five practices cholesterol concentration was measured only in a random three quarters of families, as a substudy to evaluate the impact of cholesterol testing. Families allocated to no measurement of cholesterol do not appear in the results

presented here. The results for this substudy will be reported separately.

LIFESTYLE COUNSELLING AND FOLLOW UP IN
INTERVENTION GROUP

By means of a coronary risk score[16] derived from the intermediate score of the British regional heart study[17] based on both modifiable and unmodifiable risk factors, subjects were told which decile of the distribution of risk for coronary heart disease they were in relative to other men (or women) of the same age. Those who reported a history of coronary heart disease or chest pain on exercise were automatically placed in the top decile of risk. The risk score was recorded in a booklet, "Your passport to health," in which personally negotiated lifestyle changes in relation to smoking, weight, healthy eating, alcohol consumption, and exercise could be documented. When appropriate, Health Education Authority pamphlets on each of these subjects were provided. The frequency of follow up visits was determined by both the coronary risk score and individual risk factors. Adults (either partner) in the top quintile of the risk distribution were offered follow up every two months, those in the fourth quintile every three months, those in the third quintile every four months, those in the second quintile every six months, and those in the bottom quintile at one year. People with individual high risk factors—current cigarette smokers and those with a body mass index ≥ 25, diastolic blood pressure ≥ 90 mm Hg, cholesterol concentration ≥ 6.5 mmol/l, or random glucose concentration ≥ 7 mmol/l—were also invited to reattend every month for up to three months. Patients with glucose concentration ≥ 10 mmol/l or diastolic pressure ≥ 115 mm Hg on any occasion were referred to their general practitioner, as were those with cholesterol concentration ≥ 6.5 mmol/l or diastolic pressure ≥ 100 mm Hg sustained for three months.

DATA MONITORING AND QUALITY ASSURANCE

Quality of data collection was assured by a series of routine checks of nurse records (JY), by a weekly review of computer disks (YK), by weekly quality assurance returns for cholesterol and glucose concentrations (CLG, RC) organised by the Wolfson Research Laboratories, and by routine data monitoring (SP). During the one year follow up these processes showed that one nurse in an intervention practice in one of the 14 towns originally included in the study had departed from a number of protocol requirements A complete audit of the one year rescreening results in that practice showed inconsistencies between families attending and data recorded, which cast doubt on the reliability of this information. Before the main one year analyses were undertaken the executive committee decided, without sight of the data recorded, to discard all data from this intervention practice and therefore also to discard all data from the comparison practice in the same town. The statistical analyses in this report are thus based on 26 general practices from 13 towns (fig 2).

STATISTICAL METHODS

The protocol defined the main statistical comparison of risk factors to be between the intervention group rescreened at one year and the concurrently screened external comparison group. The intervention group was also compared, however, with the internal comparison group taken from the same practice. Because this latter comparison is not affected by variability between different practices it was expected to be more precise, although any effect might be diluted by some transfer of effect from the intervention to the comparison group within the same practice. The numbers of general practices and subjects recruited to the study

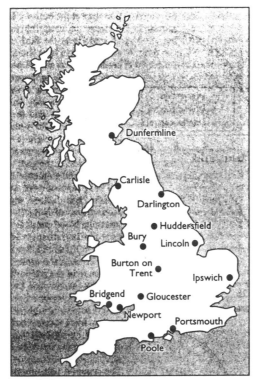

FIG 2—*Study towns*

were chosen on the basis of published information on variability of risk factors between and within different practices[18] so that the mean difference between the intervention group and external comparison group was anticipated to have a standard error of 0·05 mmol/l for blood cholesterol concentration and 2·0 mm Hg for systolic blood pressure. The principal outcome measured was defined as the Dundee risk score, an overall measure of modifiable coronary risk which depends on serum cholesterol concentration, systolic blood pressure, and previous and current smoking habit.[15] The distribution and means of individual risk factors were compared as well as the proportions of subjects with values greater than prespecified cut

off points—namely, serum cholesterol concentration ≥8·0 mmol/l, diastolic blood pressure ≥100 mm Hg, body mass index ≥30, and random blood glucose concentration ≥10 mmol/l.

For each risk factor the differences in means or proportions between intervention and comparison groups were calculated separately in each town, together with standard errors. These differences were then pooled across the 13 towns using a random effects meta-analysis.[19] The estimated difference derived is an approximately unweighted average of the differences in each town, and the standard error or confidence interval presented takes into account sources of variation between and within towns.[20] Our results are based on the man (aged 40-59 at selection) from each family recruited and on his partner, regardless of her age. The Dundee risk score was designed only for subjects aged 35-64, however, and so a small proportion of women were excluded from this analysis. Few values for risk factors were missing (indicated in the footnotes to tables as appropriate). Because age was well balanced between the intervention and comparison groups (see table I) adjustments for age had only minimal effect and so unadjusted results are presented.

TABLE I—*Numbers of subjects, mean ages, and mean percentage reduction in risk of coronary heart disease in intervention group at one year compared with external and internal comparison groups*

Group	No of subjects*	Mean age (SD) (years)	Percentage reduction in risk† in intervention group (95% confidence interval)
		Men	
Intervention	1767	51·5 (5·7)	
Comparison:			
External	3519	51·5 (5·7)	16·1 (10·9 to 21·1)
Internal	2174	51·6 (5·8)	17·6 (14·0 to 21·1)
		Women	
Intervention	1217	49·1 (6·8)	
Comparison:			
External	2393	49·0 (7·1)	15·7 (7·4 to 23·3)
Internal	1402	49·0 (6·8)	13·2 (7·3 to 18·6)

*Excluding those randomised to no measurement of cholesterol concentration (202 men and 150 women) in the cholesterol/no cholesterol substudy.
†Odds of coronary heart disease calculated from the Dundee risk score (1), based on systolic blood pressure, cholesterol concentration, and smoking habit with adjustments for age and sex. Not calculated for 16 men and 12 women because of missing blood pressure or cholesterol measurements and for a further 143 women because they were not aged 35-64.

Results

A total of 14 086 households were approached; 8605 households were represented by one or more adult members, giving a crude household response rate of 61%. After adjustment of the denominator for "ghosts" (patients on the practice lists who had died or left the practice; from a survey of non-responders we estimated the proportion of ghosts to be at least 16%), the true response rate was 73%. Crude (and adjusted) household response rates for the intervention and internal and external comparison groups were 57% (68%) (2373/4158); 62% (73%) (2342/3798); and 63% (76%) (3890/6130) respectively. Similar numbers of participants were recruited to the intervention and internal comparison groups (fig 1), but substantially more were recruited to the external comparison group because the time taken to see each family was shorter. At one year the reattendance rate of men and women in the intervention group was 88% (1969/2246) and 85% (1367/1604) respectively. At this point the age of the men in the intervention and internal and external comparison groups was between 40 and 61 (because of the selection criteria of the study), and 93% of the women were aged 35-59. The mean ages of the men and women were almost identical in all three groups. A total of 7460 men and 5012 women are included in this report.

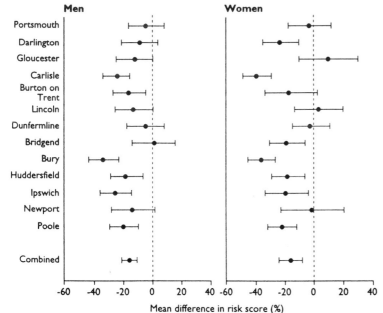

FIG 3—*Mean differences in Dundee risk score (intervention group minus external comparison group) with bars showing 95% confidence intervals for each of the 13 towns, and combined overall, for men and women separately*

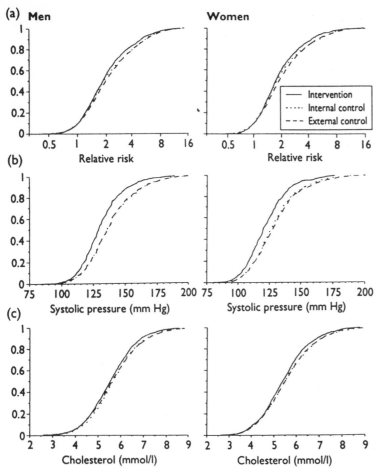

FIG 4—*Cumulative relative frequency distribution for relative risk (derived from the Dundee risk score), systolic blood pressure, and blood cholesterol concentration in intervention and comparison groups for men and women separately*

DUNDEE RISK SCORE

The Dundee risk score was approximately 16% lower at one year in the intervention group compared with either the external or internal comparison group (table I). The overall difference in mean risk score was similar in men and women but seemed to be rather more consistent across the 13 towns for men (fig 3). The distribution of risk scores shows that the difference was greatest at the top (high risk) end of the distribution (fig 4a), as the horizontal difference between the curves was greatest at high values. The risk factors did not contribute equally. For example, of the observed 16% lower risk score in men (as compared with the external comparison group), 7% was attributable to blood pressure, 5% to smoking, and 4% to cholesterol.

CARDIOVASCULAR RISK FACTORS

Individual differences in risk factors were similar in men and women, with both comparison groups giving consistent results (table II). In the intervention group at one year reported cigarette smoking among returners was lower by about 4%, systolic blood pressure by an average of 7 mm Hg and diastolic pressure by 3 mm Hg, weight by an average of about 1 kg, and cholesterol concentration by an average of about 0·1 mmol/l. For the latter, the standard errors were sufficiently large to include the possibility of no effect in women. There was no discernible shift in median random blood glucose concentrations.

The differences in the distributions of systolic blood pressure and serum cholesterol concentration are shown in figure 4 (b and c). There was a consistent tendency for greater changes at the top of the distribu-

tion than at the bottom. For example, for systolic blood pressure in men the average difference was about 10 mm Hg at the 80th centile of the distribution and about 5 mm Hg at the 20th centile. This is shown for predetermined cut off points for individual risk factors in table III. The proportion of subjects at the top end of the distributions is lower in the intervention group (except for glucose) and conversely the proportion towards the low end in the same group is increased. The differences in weight were not attributable to imbalance in height as body mass index (weight/height²) was also lower in the intervention group compared with the comparison groups by about 0·4 in both men and women.

The proportion of patients with high levels of specific risk factors are shown in table IV. The proportions of subjects with high blood pressure (diastolic blood pressure ≥ 100 mm Hg), high cholesterol concentration (≥ 8·0 mmol/l), or high body mass index (≥ 30) were lower in the intervention group than in the comparison group, but there was no discernible difference in the proportions with high random blood glucose concentration (≥ 10·0 mmol/l).

The lower reported prevalence of cigarette smoking among returners in the intervention group was accompanied by a correspondingly greater proportion of reported ex-cigarette smokers, while the proportions of cigar or pipe smokers and lifelong non-smokers were similar in the intervention and comparison groups. The reported consumption of cigarettes among cigarette smokers was slightly lower in the intervention group. For example, in men the reported average consumption was 16·8 cigarettes a day compared with 18·9 and 19·3 cigarettes a day in the external and internal comparison groups respectively. The corresponding proportions of male cigarette smokers reporting smoking 20 or more cigarettes a day were 46%, 59%, and 57% respectively. Self reported smoking habit may be biased, and breath carbon monoxide concentrations were measured in the inter-

TABLE II—*Differences in risk factors for coronary heart disease between intervention group at one year and external and internal comparison groups*

Group	Men		Women	
	Crude value*	Pooled difference (SE)†	Crude value*	Pooled difference (SE)†
	Smoking prevalence (% of subjects)			
Intervention	19·1		17·7	
Comparison:				
External	22·8	−4·1 (1·8)	21·2	−3·5 (2·1)
Internal	23·0	−4·1 (1·3)	21·5	−2·9 (1·5)
	Mean blood cholesterol (mmol/l)			
Intervention	5·58		5·48	
Comparison:				
External	5·69	−0·12 (0·06)	5·61	−0·12 (0·09)
Internal	5·72	−0·13 (0·03)	5·60	−0·09 (0·07)
	Mean systolic pressure (mm Hg)			
Intervention	131·6		123·2	
Comparison:				
External	138·8	−7·5 (1·2)	130·8	−7·7 (1·4)
Internal	139·0	−7·3 (0·8)	129·6	−6·2 (0·9)
	Mean diastolic pressure (mm Hg)			
Intervention	83·3		78·6	
Comparison:				
External	85·5	−2·5 (1·0)	80·7	−2·5 (0·9)
Internal	86·6	−3·5 (0·4)	81·3	−3·0 (0·4)
	Mean weight (kg)			
Intervention	79·55		66·06	
Comparison:				
External	80·70	−1·17 (0·36)	66·83	−1·09 (0·42)
Internal	80·76	−1·18 (0·43)	66·73	−0·74 (0·54)
	Median blood glucose (mmol/l)			
Intervention	5·54		5·50	
Comparison:				
External	5·56	−0·03 (0·08)	5·40	0·10 (0·09)
Internal	5·64	−0·11 (0·05)	5·49	0·01 (0·04)

*Calculated without regard to pairings within towns.
†Differences calculated for each town separately and then pooled over 13 towns. Pooled differences are therefore not exactly equal to differences in crude values.

vention and internal comparison groups. Among male reported ex-smokers of cigarettes who were not currently smoking pipe or cigars the proportion of men with carbon monoxide ⩾10 ppm was 1·1% in the intervention group and 0·7% in the internal comparison group; the corresponding figures for women were 0·4% and 0·5%.

HIGH BLOOD PRESSURE, HIGH BLOOD CHOLESTEROL CONCENTRATION, DIABETES, AND CORONARY HEART DISEASE

The numbers of men and women referred to their general practitioners by the nurses with very high or sustained high individual risk factor values, expressed as a proportion of the total population screened, were respectively: blood pressure (diastolic ⩾90 mm Hg) 2% (39/2246) and 1% (14/1604); cholesterol (⩾6·5 mmol/l) 5% (102/2011) and 5% (68/1425); and glucose concentration (⩾7 mmol/l) 3% (60/2246) and 1% (13/1604). At one year the proportions with reported high blood pressure and a high cholesterol concentration were substantially higher in the intervention group than in the comparison groups in both men and women, and the proportion with reported diabetes was slightly higher in the intervention group

TABLE III—*Percentages of men and women at one year with coronary risk factors within the specified ranges in intervention and external and internal comparison groups*

	Men			Women		
	Intervention	External comparison	Internal comparison	Intervention	External comparison	Internal comparison
Blood cholesterol (mmol/l):						
<6·5	82	77	78	84	79	78
6·5-7·9	16	20	19	14	18	18
⩾8·0	2	3	3	2	3	4
Diastolic pressure (mm Hg):						
<90	72	65	62	85	80	79
90-99	21	24	25	11	15	16
100-114	7	10	11	3	4	4
⩾115	0	1	1	0	1	0
Body mass index (kg/m²):						
<20·0	2	2	1	5	4	5
20·0-24·9	38	34	33	54	48	49
25·0-29·9	48	50	52	29	34	33
30·0-34·9	11	11	12	9	10	10
⩾35·0	1	3	2	3	4	4
Blood glucose (mmol/l):						
<7·0	87	85	85	90	93	90
7·0-9·9	11	13	13	9	7	9
⩾10·0	2	2	2	1	1	1

TABLE IV—*Percentages (numbers) of men and women with high serum cholesterol concentration, diastolic pressure, body mass index, and blood glucose concentration at one year in intervention groups compared with external and internal comparison groups*

	Men		Women	
Group	Crude prevalence (%)*	Pooled difference (SE)†	Crude prevalence (%)*	Pooled difference (SE)†
	Blood cholesterol ⩾8·0 mmol/l			
Intervention	2·0 (35)		2·1 (25)	
Comparison:				
External	3·4 (119)	-1·5 (0·8)	2·9 (69)	-1·1 (0·5)
Internal	2·7 (58)	-1·2 (0·4)	3·7 (52)	-1·7 (0·7)
	Diastolic pressure ⩾100 mm Hg			
Intervention	7·0 (124)		3·5 (43)	
Comparison:				
External	11·2 (393)	-4·6 (1·4)	5·2 (125)	-2·2 (1·1)
Internal	12·5 (272)	-5·3 (1·1)	4·9 (68)	-1·4 (0·9)
	Body mass index ⩾30 kg/m²			
Intervention	12·0 (212)		12·4 (151)	
Comparison:				
External	13·7 (481)	-1·8 (1·3)	14·1 (337)	-2·2 (1·5)
Internal	13·6 (296)	-1·7 (1·2)	13·8 (193)	-1·7 (1·3)
	Blood glucose ⩾10·0 mmol/l			
Intervention	2·3 (40)		1·0 (12)	
Comparison:				
External	2·2 (76)	-0·1 (0·4)	0·5 (12)	0·3 (0·3)
Internal	2·3 (50)	0·1 (0·4)	0·8 (11)	0·2 (0·4)

*Calculated without regard to pairings within towns.
†Differences calculated for each town separately and then pooled over 13 towns. Pooled differences are therefore not exactly equal to differences in crude values.

TABLE V—*Percentages (numbers) of subjects at one year who reported having been diagnosed as having coronary heart disease (angina, coronary artery bypass graft, or heart attack), diabetes, high blood pressure, or high cholesterol concentration*

	Men		Women	
Group	Crude prevalence (%)*	Pooled difference (SE)†	Crude prevalence (%)*	Pooled difference (SE)†
	Coronary heart disease			
Intervention	5·9 (105)		1·9 (23)	
Comparison:				
External	6·5 (227)	-0·6 (0·9)	1·3 (31)	0·3 (0·4)
Internal	5·5 (119)	0·29 (0·9)	1·1 (16)	0·5 (0·5)
	Diabetes			
Intervention	3·3 (59)		1·2 (15)	
Comparison:				
External	2·4 (85)	0·6 (0·5	0·9 (22)	0·1 (0·3)
Internal	1·7 (38)	1·5 (0·5)	1·1 (16)	0·2 (0·4)
	High blood pressure			
Intervention	17·1 (302)		16·2 (197)	
Comparison:				
External	13·5 (474)	3·2 (1·6)	11·5 (275)	4·1 (2·3)
Internal	14·8 (322)	2·4 (1·2)	13·0 (182)	3·7 (1·4)
	High cholesterol			
Intervention	14·0 (247)		9·7 (118)	
Comparison:				
External	9·5 (336)	4·0 (1·7)	5·1 (123)	4·0 (1·2)
Internal	6·9 (150)	66 (1·5)	3·8 (53)	5·7 (1·3)

*Calculated without regard to pairings within towns.
†Differences calculated for each town separately and then pooled over 13 towns. Pooled differences are therefore not exactly equal to differences in crude values.

in men (table V). In the whole population there was no reported difference in the proportions of patients taking drugs to lower blood pressure or cholesterol concentrations or for diabetes between the intervention and comparison groups. The proportions of patients at one year with reported coronary heart disease (angina, heart attack, coronary artery surgery) were similar in intervention and comparison groups.

NON-RETURNERS

The intervention group necessarily comprised those who were recruited to the study one year before and who also returned at one year, while for the comparison groups the one year point represented their first screening visit. Table VI shows the effect of the potential bias introduced by non-returners by showing the mean risk factor values at initial recruitment in the intervention group among those who returned at one year (comprising 88% of men and 85% of women) compared with those who did not. There was a much greater prevalence of cigarette smoking among those who did not return compared with those who did. Weight was on average slightly higher among the non-returners, but no other measured risk factor showed clear differences. There was, however, generally a slightly higher prevalence of coronary heart disease and diagnosed diabetes, reported high blood pressure, and high blood cholesterol concentration among those who returned compared with those who did not.

Discussion

In this national trial of a nurse led cardiovascular screening and lifestyle intervention in general practice the overall Dundee risk score was 16% lower after intervention. This lower risk score was consistent when comparing the intervention group with either the external or internal comparison groups and was similar for both men and women. A lower blood pressure accounted for almost half of the observed lower risk, with smoking accounting for a third and cholesterol concentration for about a quarter. The true difference in coronary risk, however, is actually less because differences in smoking are considerably smaller when the smoking habits of those who did not return at one year are taken into account, and the lower blood pressure is likely to be due partly to acclimatisation to

TABLE VI—*Initial risk factor values among subjects on recruitment to intervention group according to whether they returned at one year*

	Men			Women		
	Returned at one year	Did not return at one year	Pooled difference (SE)*	Returned at one year	Did not return at one year	Pooled difference (%)*
No (%) of subjects	1767 (88)	244 (12)		1217 (85)	208 (15)	
Mean age (years)	50·5	49·9	0·7 (0·5)	48·2	47·7	0·4 (0·5)
% Of subjects with:						
Coronary heart disease	5·4	3·3	3·3 (1·3)	1·3	0·5	0·8 (1·2)
Diabetes	2·3	1·2	1·7 (1·1)	0·9	0·5	0·9 (1·2)
High blood pressure	14·5	16·4	0·8 (2·7)	14·5	9·6	6·6 (2·4)
High cholesterol	8·3	4·1	5·9 (1·4)	3·8	2·4	1·7 (1·3)
No (%) of subjects who smoked cigarettes	22·2	41·8	-19·0 (3·4)	19·4	38·9	-18·1 (4·5)
Mean blood cholesterol (mmol/l)	5·67	5·60	0·03 (0·08)	5·50	5·53	-0·01 (0·11)
Mean blood pressure (mm Hg):						
Systolic	138·9	140·7	-0·9 (1·5)	129·4	129·4	1·8 (1·5)
Diastolic	87·1	88·6	-1·2 (0·8)	81·6	82·1	0·1 (0·8)
Mean weight (kg)	79·9	81·7	-1·7 (0·8)	65·9	68·1	-1·9 (0·9)
Median blood glucose (mmol/l)	5·42	5·45	0·02 (0·08)	5·27	5·30	0·06 (0·07)

*Differences calculated for each town separately and then pooled over 13 towns. Pooled differences are therefore not exactly equal to difference in two values.

measurement in the intervention group. We now consider what reduction in the risk of coronary events could be anticipated from the results of this trial.

BIASES IN ASSESSING RISK FACTORS

The lower smoking prevalence observed in the intervention group is biased by two factors. Firstly, a proportion of those recruited at baseline in the intervention practices did not return at one year (12% of men and 15% of women) and the prevalence of smoking at baseline among these non-returners was more than twice as high in both men and women. Secondly, those returning in the intervention group at one year may also have underreported cigarette smoking, as found in other studies.[5-8] Measurement of breath carbon monoxide concentration in our study provided little direct evidence of differential misreporting of smoking habits between the intervention and internal comparison group but is not a very reliable validator of reported smoking habit because of short half life and non-specificity. If it is assumed that the intervention group participants seen at baseline who did not return at one year had not altered their smoking habit, and among the reported ex-cigarette smokers those with a breath carbon monoxide concentration of over 10 ppm were in fact still smoking cigarettes, the observed reduction in the crude proportion of cigarette smokers of 3·9% in men compared with the internal comparison group should be adjusted to 1·0%, and for women the 3·8% difference should be adjusted to 0·7%. The difference in prevalence of smoking between returners and non-returners clearly considerably weakens the evidence for a true reduction in cigarette smoking in the intervention group.

The observed lower blood pressure may also not be entirely true as it could be partly due to the acclimatisation or habituation effect with repeated measurements over time. This effect may be due to lower stress associated with knowing both the person taking the blood pressure and the procedures of screening. To what extent the reduction in blood pressure associated with intervention in this study could be due to such acclimatisation is difficult to assess. Directly comparable data in a population (as opposed to a group with high blood pressure, such as in a hypertension trial, which is also subject to regression to the mean) is needed for this evaluation. Repeated blood pressure measurements in population groups over a three week period in the Intersalt study showed on average a reduction of 3·5 mm Hg systolic and 1·5 mm Hg diastolic in men and almost identical results in women (P Elliot, personal communication). These data suggest, albeit indirectly, that acclimatisation may

explain about half the reduction in blood pressure observed in this study.

The results for cholesterol are not open to these biases, but the average reductions were only about 0·1 mmol/l. Like the lower blood pressure this difference in cholesterol concentration will be partly due to the true difference in weight, about 1 kg lower in the intervention group.

If reductions of 0·1 mmol/l in blood cholesterol and 1·5 mm Hg in diastolic blood pressure (half that observed), but no reduction in cigarette smoking, were therefore attributed to the screening and intervention programme in this study, what effect would this have on the risk of coronary events? Using information from reviews of the effects of blood pressure[21] and cholesterol[22] on the risk of coronary heart disease (which allow for the effect of regression dilution bias) and making the crucial and untested assumption that the changes in risk factors would be maintained long term, we estimate the long term proportionate reduction in coronary heart disease risk to be 12%. This risk reduction was achieved by changes in lifestyle as there was no difference at one year in the use of drugs to lower blood pressure and cholesterol concentration between the intervention and comparison groups. If the screening and intervention programme used in this trial were implemented in the same way by every general practice in the country, and if such programmes achieved the same reductions in risk factors (which were then maintained long term), and if this was translated into prevention of myocardial infarction and saving of lives the overall impact on the population burden of coronary heart disease would be small. A risk reduction of 12% in men aged 40-59 participating in the programme would potentially prevent 788 myocardial infarctions and 853 deaths from coronary heart disease each year, which is about 8% of all such events in British men of this age.

APPLICABILITY OF INTERVENTION

The intervention evaluated in this study was designed to use the maximum resources currently available to general practice. The trial used an innovative approach to cardiovascular screening by offering screening to families rather than individual people because it seemed more likely that changes in lifestyle in relation to smoking habit, eating, and exercise would occur if the whole household participated.[23] This family approach, with its initial one and a half hour screening interview for each couple, is very different from the original government sponsored health promotion clincs based on payment for seeing 10 patients in one hour. It bears more similarities to the risk related team approach recommended in the new health promotion package for primary care,[2] but with a full time trained nurse dedicated to the screening and follow up programme and its focus on families rather than individual people our intervention is likely to exceed in its intensity all but that of the most dedicated practice teams elsewhere. The extent to which the nurses were incorporated into an effective primary care team in each practice was highly variable, and leading lifestyle groups was beyond the nurses' resources, although families were encouraged to seek help in other ways—for example, from Weight Watchers. The nurses were fully occupied with the demands of screening, counselling, and following up an average of 183 families (about 296 individuals) during the year. This represented about a sixth of the total practice population potentially eligible for this programme. So a practice with a list size of 1000 men (aged 40-59) that wanted to implement this family based screening and intervention programme would require at least four full time nurses to screen and interview men and their partners over a period of 18 months.

The nurses were trained to facilitate healthy behavioural changes in families using client centred counselling rather than simply giving advice, and they encouraged all families to make the same healthy lifestyle choices regardless of their level of risk. The intensity of nursing intervention, in relation to the family's smoking, dietary, and exercise habits and their subsequent follow up, was determined by the highest coronary risk score in that family, as well as by single risk factors alone. This reflected our belief that rational use of resources to encourage changes in lifestyle should be in proportion to the overall level of risk. Family members were told their risk relative to other men and women of their own age and this avoided classifying people's results as normal or abnormal according to the traditional model of medical screening. This approach was reflected in the change in risk that was achieved; it was greatest at the top (high risk) end of the distribution. Those with high values for one or more individual risk factors, such as blood pressure, were followed up in the traditional way with monthly review as well, and some were then referred to their general practitioner for consideration of drug treatment. However, there was in fact no difference at one year in the overall prevalence of drug treatment between the intervention and comparison groups.

The only randomised controlled trial of multiphasic screening previously reported from general practice was undertaken in two large group practices in south London and based on 3297 middle-aged men and women.[4] The response rate to the initial screening was 73% and to a second screening two years later was 65·5%. Multiphasic screenings included height, weight, blood pressure, smoking, and serum cholesterol concentration but no formal intervention was offered. Over the subsequent nine years there were no significant differences in morbidity or mortality between those screened and not screened. The power of this study to detect major differences in incidence of and mortality from cardiovascular disease was weak, and the trial result should be considered inconclusive for this end point.

Our systematic approach to cardiovascular screening and lifestyle intervention in general practice in this trial did not reach everybody in the population. Though most adults in the age range we studied are registered with a general practitioner, about 40% of those who were potentially eligible to attend did not do so. Some of these non-responders are ghosts on the practice lists. To estimate the impact of any intervention on the population as a whole the number and characteristics of non-responders need to be measured. Other surveys of non-responders in general practice have found a higher prevalence of smoking, obesity, and alcohol consumption compared with those who attend.[24 25] In our study the household response rate after allowing for ghosts was 73%, so about a quarter of the population did not participate. In addition, of those who came to the initial baseline screening, 12% of men and 15% of women did not return at one year despite every effort by the nurses to maximise response rates. These non-returners were twice as likely to be cigarette smokers and were more overweight than returners but interestingly showed a slightly lower prevalence of diagnosed disease. Thus it appears those who come for screening and then participate in an intervention programme over one year contain both a disproportionately larger number of people with lower risk factors and a slightly higher proportion of patients with diagnosed hypertension, hypercholesterolaemia, diabetes, or overt coronary heart disease.

SUMMARY

The results of this large national trial, which is one of two studies evaluating nurse led progrmmes of cardio-

Clinical implications

- A national general practice nurse led cardiovascular screening and lifestyle intervention programme reached 73% of eligible families and maintained contact with 88% of men and 85% of women over one year
- After one year reported cigarette smoking was lower by about 4%, weight by 1 kg, systolic pressure by 7 mm Hg, diastolic pressure by 3 mm Hg, and cholesterol concentration by 0·1 mmol/l on average
- Smoking prevalence, however, was twice as high in those who did not return at one year compared with those who did
- This intensive family centred programme achieved at most an overall 12% reduction in coronary risk (Dundee risk score), similar in both men and women
- The voluntary health promotion package in primary care cannot be justified, in its present form, by these results, and alternative preventive strategies need to be developed and evaluated

vascular screening and lifestyle intervention in general practice,[26] found slightly lower weight, blood pressure, and blood cholesterol concentration at one year in the intervention group. Whether these small reductions could be sustained long term is not known, but even if they were they would correspond only to a 12% lower risk of coronary heart disease events. As this lower risk was achieved with a family based programme led by nurses trained in learner centred techniques, and with intensive follow up in relation to overall coronary heart disease risk, as well as individual risk factors, the government sponsored health promotion clinic sessions with no financial commitment to follow up, would probably have achieved considerably less and possibly no change at all. Whether the new health promotion package for general practice, which encourages a more opportunistic approach to screening the population reflecting the reiterative contact of patients with the primary care team, will achieve useful reductions in risk must remain in considerable doubt and cannot be justified in its present form from the results of this trial. Other options might include focusing limited primary care resources on high risk patients—for example, those with hypertension, hyperlipidaemia, diabetes, and established coronary heart disease. Whatever new approaches are advocated this trial emphasises the need for, and shows the feasibility of, rigorous scientific evaluation to measure the impact of such strategies in the future. Clearly, primary care alone cannot provide a population approach to reducing cardiovascular risk, and the government, in aiming to reduce the prevalence of risk factors, will also need to put in place more effective public health policies on tobacco control and healthy eating.

The family heart study was coordinated by Preventive Cardiology, Medicine and Primary Medical Care, University of Southampton; the Medical Statistics Unit, London School of Hygiene and Tropical Medicine; and the Wolfson Research Laboratories, University of Birmingham. Members of the executive committee are D A Wood (chair), C Coles, R Cramb, G Davies, P Durrington, A-L Kinmonth, Y Kok, C Le Guen, T Marteau, A O'Dwyer, S M D Pyke, D W Steele, S G Thompson, and J Yarwood (secretary: C M Bicknell).

We thank the staff of the general practices and their patients, on whom the results presented in the present paper are based, and the family heart study nurses: N Credland, L

Mackenzie, S Field, K Probert, J Holloway, C Hill, L Kyle, D Howkins, C May, J Waywell, J May, S Armstrong, L McMurray, W Whitman, H Norris, K McElhone, K Pasquill-Taylor, B Kamal, J Probert, V Ferbrache, R Travis, D Sender, S Williams, H Hawes, S Glenister, J Collins, V Kemp. We acknowledge the help of the participating family health service authorities in England (Bury; Cumbria; Dorset; Durham; Gloucestershire; Hampshire; Kirklees; Lincolnshire; Staffordshire; and Suffolk) and Wales (Gwent and Mid Glamorgan) and of Fife Health Board in Scotland; Boehringer Mannheim UK; and additional members of the steering committee (P Durrington (chair), J Betteridge, M Buxton, J Garrow, M Marmot, A Maryon-Davis, J McKenzie, V Patten, S J Pocock, L Ritchie, and J Young).

The study was funded by the Family Heart Association with an educational grant from Merck Sharp and Dohme, the family health service authorities and Fife Health Board, Boehringer Mannheim UK, Wessex Regional Health Authority, the Health Education Authority, the Scottish Home and Health Department, and the Department of Health.

1 Department of Health. *The health of the nation: a strategy for health in England.* London: HMSO, 1992.
2 General Medical Services Committee. The new health promotion package. London: British Medical Association, 1993.
3 Fullard E, Fowler G, Gray M. Promoting prevention in primary care: controlled trial of low technology, low cost approach. *BMJ* 1987; 294: 1080-2.
4 South-East London Screening Study Group. A controlled trial of multiphasic screening in middle-age: results of the south-east London screening study. *Int J Epidemiol* 1977;6:357-63.
5 Jamrozik K, Vessey M, Fowler G, Wald N, Parker G, Vunakis HV. Controlled trial of three different antismoking interventions in general practice. *BMJ* 1984;288:1449-503.
6 Richmond RL, Austin A, Webster IW. Three year evaluation of a programme by general practitioners to help patients to stop smoking. *BMJ* 1986;292:803-6.
7 Imperial Cancer Research Fund General Practice Research Group. Effectiveness of a nicotine patch in helping people stop smoking: results of a randomised trial in general practice. *BMJ* 1993;306:1304-8.
8 Russell MAH, Stapleton JA, Feyerabend C, Wiseman SM, Gustavsson G,

9 Medical Research Council Working Party. MRC trial of treatment of mild hypertension: principal results. *BMJ* 1985;291:97-104.
10 Mant D, McKinlay C, Fuller A, Randall T, Fullard EM, Muir J. Three year follow up of patients with raised blood pressure identified at health checks in general practice. *BMJ* 1989;298:1360-2.
11 Ritchie LD, Currie AM. Blood pressure recording by general practitioners in north-east Scotland. *BMJ* 1983;286:107-9.
12 Kurji KH, Haines AP. Detection and management of hypertension in general practices in north west London. *BMJ* 1984;288:903-7.
13 Hayes TM, Harries J. Randomised controlled trial of routine hospital clinic care versus routine general practice care for type II diabetics. *BMJ* 1984;289:728-30.
14 Family Heart Study Group. British family heart study: its design and method, and prevalence of cardiovascular risk factors. *Br J Gen Pract* 1994;44:62-7.
15 Tunstall-Pedoe H. The Dundee coronary risk-disk for management of change in risk factors. *BMJ* 1991;303:744-7.
16 Thompson SG, Pyke SDM, Wood DA on behalf of the British Family Heart Study. Using a coronary risk score for screening and intervention in general practice. *Health Trends* (in press).
17 Shaper AG, Pocock SJ, Phillips AN, Walker M. A scoring system to identify men at high risk of a heart attack. *Health Trends* 1987;19:37-9.
18 Shaper AG, Pocock SJ, Walker M, Cohen NM, Wale CJ, Thomson AG. British regional heart study: cardiovascular risk factors in middle-aged men in 24 towns. *BMJ* 1981;283:179-86.
19 DerSimonian R, Laird N. Meta-analysis in clinical trials. *Controlled Clin Trials* 1986;7:177-8.
20 Donner A, Donald A. Analysis of data arising from a stratified design with the cluster as unit of randomization. *Stat Med* 1987;6:43-52.
21 MacMahon S, Peto R, Cutler J, Collins R, Sorlie P, Neaton J, *et al.* Blood pressure, stroke, and coronary heart disease. *Lancet* 1990;335:765-74.
22 Law MR, Wald NJ, Thompson SG. By how much and how quickly does serum cholesterol reduction lower the risk of ischaemic heart disease? *BMJ* (in press).
23 Kolonel LN, Lee J. Husband-wife correspondence in smoking, drinking, and dietary habits. *American Journal of Clinical Nutrition* 1981;34:99-104.
24 Pill R, French J, Harding K, Stott N. Invitation to attend a health check in a general practice setting: comparison of attenders and non-attenders. *J R Coll Gen Pract* 1988;38:53-6.
25 Difford F, Telling JP, Davies KR, Fornear JE, Reading CA. Continuous opportunistic and systematic screening for hypertension with computer help: analysis of non-responders. *BMJ* 1987;294:1130-2.
26 Imperial Cancer Research Fund OXCHECK Study Group. Prevalence of risk factors for heart disease in OXCHECK trial: implications for screening in primary care. *BMJ* 1991;302:1057-60.

Sawe U, *et al.* Targeting heavy smokers in general practice: randomised controlled trial of transdermal nicotine patches. *BMJ* 1993;306:1308-12.

(Accepted 13 January 1994)

HEALTH PROMOTION INTERNATIONAL
© Oxford University Press 1993

Vol. 8, No. 4
Printed in Great Britain

Skin cancer: do early childcare centres provide protection?

MARGOT J. SCHOFIELD, ANDREW COXALL, and
ROB W. SANSON-FISHER
New South Wales Cancer Council Cancer Education Research Project, Faculty of Medicine, University of Newcastle, NSW, Australia

SUMMARY

Increasing skin cancer rates highlight the need to reduce the amount of solar exposure of young children. Children in early childcare are one potential target group for improved sun protection policy and practice. Solar protection policies and practices in 51 randomly selected early childcare centres in the Hunter Region of New South Wales, Australia were examined. Only 18% of centres had written policies and 36% of centres *unwritten policies, predominantly hat and sunscreen policies. The sun protection practices of 306 children across the 51 centres was also examined. The adoption of specific policies by the centre was not associated with increased protection of children within that centre. The need for effective implementation and maintenance strategies is highlighted.*

Key words: skin cancer; policy; early childcare

INTRODUCTION

Skin cancer is a serious and growing problem at a time when most forms of preventable cancer are declining in incidence (National Cancer Institute, 1989). The disease is increasingly seen in younger age groups, and is the most common cancer in the under-40s (Elwood *et al.*, 1988). It is estimated that 80% of skin cancers are preventable through limiting ultraviolet (UV) exposure (Stern *et al.*, 1986), and the critical period for sustaining damaging levels of sun exposure occurs during the early childhood years (Lee, 1982; Holman *et al.*, 1986). Preschool aged children are thus an important target group for sun protection interventions.

In the Australian setting, approximately 16% of preschool aged children attend government funded or commercially run early childcare centres, with about 60% of all childcare places being taken by 3–4 year olds (Australian Bureau of Statistics, 1988; Commonwealth Department of Health, Housing & Community Services,

1991). Children may enrol in these centres either five days a week or for as little as one half-day session. Early childcare centres thus have the potential to have an important impact on the level of sun exposure that children sustain through these formative years and hence on the long-term risk of developing skin cancer.

The achievement of reduced sun exposure of children in early childcare centres may well be facilitated by a structural approach involving the development of comprehensive solar protection policies for centres. Comprehensive policies have been defined as those that include policies related to increased shade provision, decreased time outdoors in the middle of the day, and the use of individual sun protection devices including hats, sun protection factor (SPF) 15+ sunscreen and sun protective clothing (NSW Cancer Council, 1991). However, the link between adoption of a specific sun protection policy and improved behavioural outcomes has not been established.

M. Schofield et al.

The first aim of the study was to investigate the prevalence of solar protection policies in a randomly selected group of early childcare centres. The second aim was to examine the relationship between adoption of hat, shade, clothing and timetabling solar protection policies and the use of appropriate hats, shade, clothing and timetabling of outdoor activities. The study also investigated perceived barriers to the implementation of solar protection practices.

METHOD

Sample

Fifty-five early childcare centres (ECCs) were randomly selected by computer generated random digits from the 216 preschools and long day care centres in the lower Hunter region of New South Wales, Australia. Four of these centres were unable to be contacted (contact rate: 93%), yielding a sample of 37 preschools and 14 long day care centres ($n = 51$, consent rate 100%). A 17-item telephone interview was administered to ECC directors in summer 1989–1990. Direct observations of six systematically selected children from each centre took place during a one hour outdoor play period, giving a sample of 306 children. Only six children per centre were chosen to give a feasible number for the observer to track, and to minimize the clustering bias that would occur by including a larger number per centre.

Measures

Policy interview

The telephone interview schedule asked whether centres had a written solar protection policy, and what types of solar protection policies and practices were used, such as hats, sunscreen, shade and timetabling. Directors were also asked whether they thought early childcare centres should have a solar protection policy, their perceived barriers to implementation of policies and the number of children enrolled.

Observed protection

At each centre, trained observers attended for an hour period closest to the middle of the day when children were normally scheduled for outdoor activity. All centres were visited once over a three-week period on sunny warm days only. From children playing outdoors, they systematic-

ally selected six children according to predetermined protocol: every third or fourth child (depending on the number outdoors) was included by scanning from left to right. Identification features were recorded to facilitate repeat observations. Observers made 10 ratings of each child at 5–6 min intervals over 1 h on five protection categories: child in sun, shade, or partial shade; amount of head protection; amount of arm, leg, and foot protection. While the amount of arm, leg and foot protection was expected to remain fairly stable over time, shade and hat protection was expected to be considerably more variable due to the nature of preschool children's play. The age and sex of observed children were also recorded.

RESULTS

All 51 early childcare centres consented. The median enrolment was 79 children per week (range 23–267), and a total of 6424 children attended the centres in a week long period, although not all attended every day. Observations were carried out only on 3–4 year old children since this age group accounts for 60% of all children in childcare and because older preschool children typically undertake more outdoor play. The median time period for direct observations was 11 a.m.–midday. The observed children were 194 (63%) 4-year-olds, and 93 (30%) 3-year-olds, 154 boys and 152 girls.

Policies

Only nine (18%) centres had a formal written solar protection policy. A further 18 (36%) centres had an unwritten policy on solar protection practices. Thus, in all, 27 centres (53%) reported having a policy: 23 centres (45%) had a hat policy, 23 centres (45%) had a sunscreen policy, 12 centres (24%) had a timetable policy, 10 centres (20%) had a clothing policy, and seven centres (14%) had a shade policy. Ninety per cent of directors of centres without a policy thought that they should have a policy.

Observed protection

A total of 34 children (11%) were observed wearing a hat on at least one occasion during the 1 h period, but only four children (1%) wore a hat for all 10 observations. A total of 303 children (99%) were observed using shade for at least one observation and 183 (60%) for more than half the

Skin protection in early childcare

Table 1: Association between specific sun protection policies and practices

	ECCs with a policy		ECCs with no policy		χ^2	d.f.	P	OR
	n	%	n	%				
Hat use	19	13.8	15	8.9	1.340	1	0.247	1.629
Shade use	19	45.2	164	62.1	3.623	1	0.057	0.504
Clothing use	30	50.0	108	43.9	0.499	1	0.480	1.278
Timetabling	11	91.7	31	79.5	Fisher's exact 2-tail P = 0.666			

observations. Only 41 (13%) were in the shade for all 10 observations. A total of 138 (45%) children had good clothing protection, defined as long sleeves rolled down and legs and feet covered for all 10 observations. A general protection score was then calculated. When protection was defined as having either hat, shade or clothing protection, 222 (73%) of children were protected at least 50% of the time, and 143 (47%) were protected all of the time. Defining protection as using either hat or shade (two common forms of policy) only 103 (34%) children were protected 50% of the time, and eight (3%) children were protected all of the time. Between 11 a.m. and 3 p.m., 84% of children spent some time outdoors (median: 1 h, range: 0–3 h).

Policy versus practice

Chi-square analyses were undertaken to test whether a hat policy was associated with hat use, a shade policy was associated with play in the shade, and a clothing policy was associated with clothing protection. The criterion level of number of observations for each form of protection was chosen by examining the distributions: hat use on at least one occasion; being in full or partial shade more than 50% of the time; having arms, legs and feet protected on all observations (see Table 1). None of the three specific policies was associated with an increase in specific solar protection behaviours related to each policy. A Fisher's Exact Test of Association between having a timetable policy and spending more than an hour in the sun between 11 a.m. and 3 p.m. also revealed no significant association (2-tail, $p = 0.666$).

Barriers

All directors were asked how likely they thought a number of potential barriers were in preventing

Table 2: Perceived barriers to solar protection in early childcare centres

Perceived barrier	Directors who think this is a likely barrier*	
	n	%
Lack of support from parents	29	56.9
Lack of outdoor shelters	32	62.7
Lack of a firm policy	23	46.0
Lack of time to implement	20	39.2
Cost	13	26.0
Lack of compliance by the child	14	27.5
Peer influence	5	9.8
Lack of support from staff	2	3.9

*Number of directors = 51.

an adequate level of solar protection of children in centres. The results are shown in Table 2.

DISCUSSION

Policies

Only 18% of early childcare centres had a written policy about sun protection for children in their care, although 53% of all centres reported some form of sun protection policy or practice. Among existing policies, there was heavy reliance on individual forms of protction such as hat and sunscreen use. While these are relatively effective forms of protection when used appropriately, they are the forms most subject to failures in implementation since they rely on individual children, parents or teachers to remember each day. Relatively little emphasis had been placed on more structural policies such as reducing exposure in the middle of the day and increasing shade. Both these methods offer the potential for

M. Schofield et al.

increased protection which is not subject to the vagaries of daily behaviour. For instance, once shade structures or trees have been put in place, they remain a stable feature of the environment which will ensure some protection regardless of individual behaviours, weather patterns or changes in staff and levels of commitment to the policy. Similarly, timetable policies offer a relatively stable change likely to influence solar exposure levels over time.

Observed protection

The findings suggest that the level of protection for children in early childcare centres is less than optimal. Only 1% of children were wearing a hat on all 10 observations, only 13% of children were in shade for all observations, only 3% of children were protected by hat or shade on all occasions, and only 16% of centres timetabled to avoid outdoor activities between 11 a.m. and 3 p.m., the time when damage is most likely to occur. Conclusions drawn from this study need to be qualified since the sample of early childcare centres was small, observations were carried out on one day only, and it is not known how representative the observed behaviours are. However, preschool directors knew the subject of the study and when observers were coming, and thus if any bias existed, it was likely to have been in the direction of higher than normal protection. Further work is needed to obtain multiple baseline measures on a larger sample of early childcare centres. Future research may also need to investigate sun protection measures over varying weather conditions since it is likely that protection may vary with the weather.

Policy versus practice

Growing interest has been shown in the potential for healthy public policy to improve the health status of communities (Ottawa Charter, 1988; Winett *et al.*, 1989; Stokols, 1992). Structural approaches to health promotion such as policy development and legislative change allow for change at multiple levels to create environments which are health promoting and which complement and reinforce individual behaviours (Winett *et al.*, 1989; Stokols, 1992). As noted by McKinlay (1975) 'One stroke of effective health legislation is equal to many separate health intervention endeavours and the cumulative efforts of innumerable health workers over long periods of time. . . .' (p. 13)

With preschool aged children this sort of approach could be particularly important since it is potentially cost-effective and it does not rely on the limited capability of such children to take responsibility for their own behaviour. However, the findings of this study suggest that policy was not associated with increased levels of sun protection. Having a policy may be a necessary but not sufficient condition for achieving solar protection. The failure to find the expected link between adoption of a policy and behaviour change may be due to a number of factors. First, the sample size of this study was small and thus any conclusions can only be tentative. Second, interpretation of the finding needs to be cautioned by the fact that most early childcare centres in this study had not developed formal written policies but reported unwritten policies. It could be that a stronger commitment to implementing sun protection practices is generated through the process of developing a formal policy statement which is accepted by both staff and parents, then undertaking careful and ongoing training of staff, and implementing adequate maintenance strategies such as award systems, regular education and prompts.

A third reason for failing to find an association between policy adoption and solar protection practices may lie in the nature of policy implementation. Model sun protection policy statements are now readily available from cancer organizations along with clearly defined strategies for encouraging their adoption by early childcare centres. Guidelines are now needed to help early childcare centres translate policy statements into practical actions. ECCs may need to focus attention particularly on adequate implementation of structural sun protection strategies. Structural changes such as timetable changes and increased outdoor shade offer potentially effective forms of protection that are currently under-utilized or inadequately implemented (Schofield *et al.*, 1991). However, if appropriately implemented, they offer a high and consistent level of protection which does not rely on variable daily patterns of behaviour. What is now needed is further research to examine the impact of particular implementation strategies to ensure stable behavioural and environmental changes specified in the policies.

ACKNOWLEDGEMENTS

This research was undertaken by the NSW Cancer Council Cancer Education Research

Project, directed by Prof. R. W. Sanson-Fisher. The views expressed are not necessarily those of the Cancer Council. The cooperation of the early childcare centres is greatly appreciated.

Address for correspondence:
The Secretary
NSW Cancer Council Cancer Education Research Project
Faculty of Medicine
University of Newcastle
Locked Bag No 10
Wallsend, NSW 2287
Australia

REFERENCES

Australian Bureau of Statistics (November 1988) *Commercial Long Day Child Care Australia*. Australian Bureau of Statistics, Canberra.

Commonwealth Department of Health, Housing & Community Services. (1991) *1991 Census of Child Care Services*. Commonwealth Department of Health, Housing & Community Services, Canberra.

Elwood, J. M., Cooke, K. R., Coombs, B. D., Cox, B., Hand, J. E. and Skegg, D. C. J. (1988) A strategy for the control of malignant melanoma in New Zealand. *New Zealand Medical Journal*, **101**, 602–604.

Holman, C. D. J., Armstrong, B. K., Heenan, P. J., Blackwell, J. B., Cumming, F. J., English, D. R., Holland, S., Kelsall, G. R. H., Matz, L. R., Rouse, I. L., Singh, A., Ten Seldam, R. E. J., Watt, J. D. and Xu, A. (1986) The causes of malignant melanoma: results from the West Australian Lions Melanoma Research Project. *Recent Results in Cancer Research*, **102**, 18–37.

Lee, J. A. H. (1982) Melanoma and exposure to sunlight. *Epidemiologic Reviews*, **4**, 110–136.

McKinlay, J. B. (1975) A case for refocusing upstream: the political economy of illness. In Enelow, A. J. and Henderson, J. B. (Eds), *Applying Behavioral Science to Cardiovascular Risk* (pp. 7–17). American Heart Association, Washington, DC.

National Cancer Institute, Division of Cancer Prevention and Control Surveillance Program. (1989) *Cancer Statistics Review 1973–1986 including a Report on the Status of Cancer Control, May 1989*. US DHHS, National Cancer Institute, Bethesda, MD, NIH Publ. No. 89-2789.

New South Wales Cancer Council. (1991) *Sunsmart Advice for Early Childhood Centres*. NSW Cancer Council, Sydney.

Ottawa Charter for Health Promotion. (1987) Ottawa Charter for Health Promotion. *Health Promotion*, **1**, iii–v.

Schofield, M. J., Tripodi, D. A., Girgis, A. and Sanson-Fisher, R. W. (1991) Solar protection issues for schools: policy, practice and recommendations. *Australian Journal of Public Health*, **15**, 135–141.

Stern, R. S., Weinstein, M. C. and Baker, S. G. (1986) Risk reduction for nonmelanoma skin cancer with childhood sunscreen use. *Archives of Dermatology*, **122**, 537–543.

Stokols, D. (1992) Establishing and maintaining healthy environment: Towards a social ecology of health promotion. *American Psychologist*, **47**, 6–22.

Winett, R. A., King, A. C., and D. G. (1989) *Health Psychology and Public Health: An Integrative Approach*. Pergamon, New York.

THE GUARDIAN
Wednesday July 20 1994

Woman accused of Abbie abduction 'could not cope after shame of losing own baby'

Report: John Mullin and Paul Myers

JULIE Kelley, the woman accused of abducting baby Abbie Humphries, had a nervous breakdown after a miscarriage last year, her father said yesterday.

Ms Kelley, aged 22, who gave up her job as a dental nurse last year because of ill health, is understood to be four months pregnant. There were suggestions last night she may have snatched Abbie, four hours old when she disappeared from the Queen's Medical Centre, Nottingham, on July 1, because she was afraid her latest pregnancy might also end in miscarriage.

Abbie was meanwhile said to be thriving since being returned to her parents on Saturday. A spokeswoman for the family said: "Abbie has again been examined by a top consultant paediatrician and is both fit and well. She has taken to the breast, putting on 8oz, regaining some but not all of her weight loss resulting from her two-week ordeal."

Ms Kelley, whose recent conduct provoked neighbours' suspicions, was yesterday receiving treatment in the hospital wing of New Hall Prison, West Yorkshire.

Her boyfriend Leigh Gilbert, aged 23, a car mechanic, said through his solicitor he believed the baby he knew as Lucy Rosalind was his own. The couple stayed with his mother, Susan, aged 43, at her home in Brendon Drive, Nottingham.

They were not available for comment yesterday and were said to have negotiated a six-figure deal to talk exclusively to a Sunday newspaper.

Eric Kelley, aged 60, flanked by his wife, Margaret, 57, said his daughter, the couple's only child, had been "ashamed" of losing after two months the baby she was expecting last year.

"Julie had a miscarriage, and then she had a nervous breakdown because she couldn't cope. She didn't come to us when she would have needed us most, and when I asked her why, she said she was too ashamed."

Mr Kelley said Julie was again pregnant, and due to give birth around Christmas. Police and social workers were unable to confirm that.

Mrs Kelley, fighting tears as the couple spoke to reporters at their home in Nottingham, said: "She told us she just wanted somebody to love ... She'd seen this baby lying on the bed, by itself, looking up at her with these big, blue eyes, and she looked at it and said to herself: 'It's my baby, that is.'

"I'd like to say how deeply sorry we are for what our daughter Julie had done. Truthfully, we are sorry. I hope the Humphries can find it in their hearts to forgive her because, truthfully, she's ill."

Michael Morris, Ms Kelley's solicitor, told Nottingham magistrates, who remanded his client in custody for her own safety on abduction charges, the full circumstances would be made clear at the trial.

Neighbours said they had seen Ms Kelley sometimes looking heavily pregnant and on other occasions her normal shape. Police secured Abbie's return following a second visit to Brendon Drive, after neighbours checked with a midwife friend whether a child had been born at home there as Ms Kelley had told them.

Nottingham's City Hospital announced yesterday that newborn babies would be electronically tagged. The £45,000 security ring, which will also include alarms and closed circuit TV cameras, will be installed in the maternity unit scheduled to open in November.

A spokesman at the Queen's Medical Centre said the hospital was still making its security plans.

JOURNAL OF INTERPROFESSIONAL CARE, VOL. 7, NO. 3, 1993

What is community mental health?

PAUL HOGGETT

Centre for Social & Economic Research, University of the West of England

Summary *Current policies regarding community mental health assume the existence of a naturally occurring community within which mental health service users can be integrated. Given that many such individuals lack a secure sense of an 'internal community' the search for a place where they can belong takes on added significance. Drawing on recent research the author indicates that the concept of naturally occurring communities is a misleading one, many different kinds of community exist and vary in terms of the way in which they handle group anxieties and respond to human differences. If policy-makers and practitioners are to avoid imposing their own definition of community upon service users then they must reconceive communities as diverse human constructions many of which are more or less temporary and improvised social phenomena.*

Key words: *Facilitating environment; fragmented community; natural community?*

Normalisation and 'community'

Consider the following extracts from the 'mission statement' concerning the Mental Illness Strategic Plan for a Midlands Health Authority:

> The service should seek to integrate its users into natural community networks. It should ensure that normal patterns of life are followed . . .

> the service should be provided near to the person's usual environment and should seek to maximise independence of its users and build on their assets and support system . . .

> within resource boundaries the Mental Health Unit will continuously seek to improve standards of care to meet our customers' expectations.

Note first of all the assumption regarding 'natural' community networks. What is a 'natural community network'? Do they exist, whatever they are? What, for that matter, is an unnatural community network? Note the assumptions that (a) such networks do exist; and (b) that people with mental health problems can be 'integrated' within them. Note also the constant resort to words such as natural, normal and usual, as if a world out there exists which enjoys such qualities. Finally, note the emphasis given to 'community' and 'independence', key words as they fall from the lips of cabinet ministers, policy makers, and the managers and professionals who populate our welfare services: words which have become self-evidently good, like sliced bread, efficiency and the Queen Mother.

The Limehouse Fields estate is a 'real' community. It is situated towards the eastern end of Stepney in Tower Hamlets. This estate contains about 700 households, mostly tenants, in a variety of tenement blocks, 'cottages' and new tower blocks. The estate, like the

Correspondence: Paul Hoggett, Centre for Social & Economic Research, Faculty of Economics & Social Science, University of the West of England, Frenchay Campus, Coldharbour Lane, Bristol BS16 1QY.

PAUL HOGGETT

neighbouring Ocean estate, is very much at the bottom of the housing ladder in the Stepney area. In other words, tenants with least bargaining power (e.g. homeless families, people coming out of institutions) tend to end up on this estate which is regarded as 'least desirable'. In the Stepney area, you can almost see a hierarchy of estates. At the very top is the Exmouth estate—modern, all-white and well provided for in terms of facilities.

A couple of years ago I was involved in a detailed study of the Limehouse Fields estate. Most of the tenants interviewed were active in the Limehouse Fields Tenants' Association. They tended to be older (mostly over forty), most of them tended to be women, and many had lived on the estate for many years. Indeed, some have lived on the estate since it was built during the second world war. Virtually everyone interviewed, with the exception of one Malaysian woman, had grown up in the area of Stepney, Poplar or Bow, i.e. they were traditional 'Eastenders' in that sense.

The tenant who said "years ago you knew everyone but now half of them, you don't know who they are" was speaking for virtually everyone interviewed. There was a unanimous view that in the old days you didn't have to keep your doors locked, old people could go out at night, gardens were left as gardens without being vandalised, people helped each other out . . . the list went on endlessly. Without being able to say whether these perceptions of the past were accurate or not, it was fairly clear that none of these things existed at the time of my study. Not even the friendly Eastend pub was much in evidence on the ground. Most of the pubs visited in the Stepney area were as desolate during the evening as the estates were that surrounded them. One woman interviewed echoed this point when saying that as a family they had stopped going to local pubs long ago. However, the old network still kept alive. She referred to a couple of clubs—the Dockers' Club and the Vaughan Club—saying that here "you're with your own, you feel like a family".

In contrast to the old days, now, it seemed, anything goes. One tenant complained of a woman below her who kept pigeons, great flocks of them that messed up her garden balcony, "she's also got a Rottweiler, yet they (i.e. the Council) do nothing". Two others, living in a quadrant which was meant to be kept free of cars, complained vociferously about tenants who vandalised road gates in order to get their cars into the quadrant. "They've had about four letters saying that they must not put cars in there. They just take no notice". They went on "The Council put the gates on, but some tenants came and broke the locks off". They continued "Dogs—we've got miles and miles of dogs here—you used to be only allowed dogs if you were on the ground floor". They added "Here, if you're a tenant, you do as you like. The Council is just not strict enough". In the same vein others complained of drugs, noise levels, prostitution, people with AIDS and so on.

Many tenants perceive an increase in the number of people from 'bins' on the estate. Two tenants referred to one woman in Dibden House who won't let council workers into her flat because she believes that they're out to get her. One added "Don't get me wrong. I'm not against them on the estate, but there is no back-up". Some tenants referred to trouble making families "white people who just don't care, couldn't be bothered". There is a certain defensiveness to many of the attitudes that tenants expressed, but not so one tenant leader who constantly referred to the 'riff-raff'. Here she is speaking about the undesirables, "it's wrong to put alco's, drug addicts and pro's among decent people. Why should we have all the rubbish?" She went on further "the Council don't care about trouble makers, as long as they pay their rent the Council is happy". Even with this tenant, however, it was possible to find a more integrated view, everything was not simply black and white, "there are dirty white people, there are good and bad in all".

Wandering around the estate, some things were quite clear. In all the tenement blocks, the balconies had little troughs which were designed, originally, for people to grow flowers outside their flats. Only the houses at the far ends of the balconies (i.e. away from the

WHAT IS COMMUNITY MENTAL HEALTH?

communal stairways) had any flowers growing out of these troughs. The reason was that everyone else who tried to grow them found them pulled up and destroyed by passers by (not just kids). The estate was very much used in a way which might be seen as a 'dump', in other words, people who could not be rehoused in more desirable areas found themselves being rehoused here. People coming out of institutions; people who'd been evicted from other areas because of being troublemakers; young, single homeless; Bangladeshi families; migrant and refugee families—a great mixing pot of different ages, cultures and lifestyles in which no common or implicit rules of behaviour had been established. The sub-cultural system that had inhabited the estate many years ago had declined to a point whereby it was unable to sustain its own organic rules of behaviour in the locality. And the Council itself had withdrawn from imposing externally held rules, other than the rule of paying the rent.

How representative Limehouse Fields is of other neighbourhoods in city areas I do not know, my guess is that although there may be some things about it which are unique it probably fairly accurately portrays the living conditions and experiences of the forgotten legion within Thatcherite society—i.e. that grouping which some on both right (Charles Murray, 1984; 1990) and left (Wilson, 1987) describe as the new underclass.

Such neighbourhoods exist on the social and political margins of our society, they can be found in most inner city areas, on many of the big outer city estates and in many of the 'rough' neighbourhoods in small towns up and down the country. Many of them were once quite homogeneous in their social composition but they have become increasingly the site where a great mixture of different groups and cultures meet and live, including people with mental health problems.

If the experience of the USA is anything to go by we should pause for thought here, for when our government speaks of 'care in the community' we should face the fact that it is probably the kind of community I have been describing here to which many people from psychiatric institutions will finally come. And, as I noted regarding the Limehouse Fields, in neighbourhoods such as these there are often no common or implicit rules of behaviour, and hence no 'normal' patterns of life if by normal we are to imply 'customary' or 'typical'.

Concepts of community

We are used to speaking of neighbourhoods like the Limehouse Fields as 'communities', for example we still tend to talk about 'inner city communities'. The dictionary definition is helpful here, 'community' is derivative of the verb to 'commune', i.e. to form an intimate association. So community tends to connote familiarity, intimacy, belongingness, etc. indeed exactly qualities which places like the Limehouse Fields don't appear to have! So, for the time being, let's think of such places as 'fragmented communities'—places which seem to lack cohesion, where different groups exist side by side cohabiting the same space but not interacting with each other, not in pubs, nor community centres, nor parks nor any other public places. Of course the point about such 'communities' is that integration into them is impossible—there is nothing to be integrated into!

There is another kind of neighbourhood which may be equally familiar. This kind of neighbourhood is much more homogeneous in its composition—everyone has a similar class background, colour or lifestyle. The degree of interaction between different groups within such neighbourhoods may be considerable but the differences here are 'acceptable' ones—age, gender and perhaps some forms of disability. For reasons which aren't entirely known, many such neighbourhoods behave as 'defended communities' (Suttles, 1972)—because they are communities based upon similarity they have come to fear difference. Integration into

PAUL HOGGETT

these communities is therefore as difficult for people with mental health problems as it is for black people.

The idea of 'community' is in fact a very slippery one—the closer you get to understanding it the less you know about it. Until very recently whenever policy makers have talked about 'communities' they have always had in mind a neighbourhood community—i.e. a sense of community derived from living in the same area. However, the term is just as appropriate to describe other forms of association based on shared characteristics other than neighbourhood—for example we speak of the Sikh community, the gay community, and so on. In a still narrower sense the term 'community' is sometimes used by those who share a particular dwelling space and lifestyle—religious and hippy communities for example.

More recently Benedict Anderson (1983) has suggested that all communities should be thought of primarily as 'imagined communities', and they should be distinguished "not by their falsity/genuineness, but by the style in which they are imagined" (p. 15). Through this simple formula Anderson neatly sidesteps the question which has tended to exercise the minds of urban sociologists for years who, when studying urban neighbourhoods such as Brixton, attempted to ascertain whether a 'real' community existed there or not. Anderson suggests that if a group of people refer to the existence of a community of which they feel themselves to be a part, and if they act on the assumption that it exists, then that community is subjectively real and therefore exists.

From this perspective a community is essentially a 'community in the mind', i.e. in the mind of the group and of the individuals belonging to that group. This enables us to understand the paradox presented by communities such as the traditional white East End one to which many of those interviewed on the Limehouse Fields estate felt that they belonged. For 'objectively' such a community barely exists any longer—the formal and informal organisation of this white community has been virtually destroyed. But despite this the community believes in its own continued existence, albeit as a beleaguered, forgotten and disadvantaged community, and it acts on the basis of this assumption—as any Bengali living in the area who has been subject to harassment will testify.

The internal community

So a community in the mind is a place inside us which may feel good or bad, fragile or strong, growing or dying, and so on. I'd like you, the reader, to hold onto this thought for a while for now I wish to turn to another body of thought altogether which is also deeply concerned with such places in the mind. Specifically I wish to turn to the work of D. W. Winnicott, the psychoanalyst and paediatrician.

Winnicott explored at great length the idea of what he termed "the facilitating environment" (1976a). His focus was the kind of human environment provided by parents, and specifically the mother, which facilitates human development in the early years of a child's life. In an article entitled "The Capacity to be Alone" (1976b) Winnicott draws our attention to a vital achievement most children accomplish during their early development. He describes this achievement in terms of a specific experience, "this experience is that of being alone, as an infant and small child, in the presence of mother" (p. 30). In other words, although the mother is physically absent she is experienced as being reliably present "even if represented for the moment by a cot or a pram or the general atmosphere of the immediate environment" (ibid.). Consistent experience of a facilitating parental environment therefore encourages the belief in the existence of a benign presence, a presence which is neither purely inside us nor outside us but rather should more properly be thought of as both inside-out and outside-in. Where no such presence exists then the child, or the adult for that matter, is condemned to a solitary life with neither the capacity to endure it nor enjoy it. They are utterly alone.

WHAT IS COMMUNITY MENTAL HEALTH?

I have tried to think of what Winnicott is saying in a slightly different way (Hoggett, 1989). The benign presence he refers to can be thought of as a kind of medium which will support us if we trust it. My feeling is that we can think of this as the primary social medium in which we are all immersed, i.e. our inter-subjectivity. To experience this medium is to experience being a part of a basic community, the benign human community. The paradox Winnicott poses is that we only experience being part of this community at the point at which we have developed the capacity to be alone. And this quality of being part of a basic human community is never entirely securely established in any of us, there is always the possibility of it being destroyed. In everyday language we refer to such episodes as (emotional) breakdown, an utterly terrifying experience of falling, drowning, disappearing, of absolute aloneness. James Glass (1989) has produced a moving book based around detailed interviews with a number of individuals who had been categorised as psychotic or borderline patients. Here is one of them, David, speaking of his experience of this absent community:

> 'Place is important to me; it's a feeling I've never had, something everyone takes for granted, a home protected by walls and love, a place you call your own. I try to find it when I'm not crazy'. (p. 33).

As the child grows this original experience of a benign or facilitating environment is reproduced in an endless series of displacements and substitutions—a corner in the child's room, a den, the home, the school, the neighbourhood—indeed all social forms, including the community, potentially have this capacity to reproduce this sense of a benign, holding environment.

The psychoanalyst Wilfred Bion talked about such a social psychological space in terms of its capacity for 'containment' (Bion, 1962; 1970), that is, its capacity to contain the fear and anxiety that we bring to life and experience from life. Again, thinking of our earliest encounters with this benign environment, symbolised perhaps in the holding and cuddling of the distressed infant by its parent, it is a place where we bring our potentially uncontainable feelings and which 'makes us better'. In contrast we might think of a malign environment as one having either no capacity to contain the feelings we bring to it or, worse, one in which the violent emotion of others is thrust into us. Indeed Hinshelwood (1989) suggests that 'affective networks' exist within all groups and institutions, networks which individuals use "as a means of passing on to others certain feeling-states, elements of identity, which they wish to disown" leading both to depersonalisation of the individual and alienation from the group. Reflecting upon group processes within therapeutic communities Hinshelwood (1987) notes that where this containing function of the group breaks down it ceases to have the capacity to contain difference, the boundaries which exist in any group between me and not-me, us and them, staff and non-staff etc. become replaced by hard impermeable barriers. And, of course, exactly the same kind of processes can be found at work in neighbourhood communities where differences based upon ethnicity, lifestyle or culture can become frozen into excluding and emotionally charged barriers.

We are now in a position to draw some of the threads of this argument together. The first thing I hope I have established is that there is no such thing as a 'natural community', all communities are constructed. Physical areas differ according to the number and variety of communities they possess, some are very homogeneous, some are very heterogeneous. Some homogeneous neighbourhoods can be places where difference arouses fear and defensive barrier formation. Such places can be thought of as 'defended (neighbourhood) communities', minorities (including those experiencing mental health problems) will tend to experience rejection and/or intrusion (e.g. verbal hostility) in such places. They are not places which facilitate development. Some heterogeneous neighbourhoods are more tolerant of differences because 'everyone is different' here in any case. However, such places often

PAUL HOGGETT

resemble fragmented communities where every group keeps to itself, cohabiting the same space but not interacting, the predominant experience here is one of isolation. Finally, some heterogeneous neighbourhoods do seem to be able to contain difference without being fragmented, a great variety of groups and communities exist in the same space and interact in a non-intrusive way. This kind of place can truly be thought of as benign or facilitating.

The lie of community

So how does all this help us to understand what is meant by the concept of 'community mental health'? I would like to examine three possible meanings. In the first instance I would like to explore the status of the concept as a form of dissimulation, that is, as a means of concealment. In the USA the de-institutionalisation movement began some time before the UK, Glass (1989) reflects on its actual effects thus: "A growing body of evidence suggests that the chronic mental patient drifts from halfway house to boarding house in the run-down sections of some large city ... what has emerged in the drearier areas of large cities is something akin to a psychological proletariat, living and (rarely) working in a social universe noticeably short on sympathy and empathy" (p. 195).

Yes, this is partly a problem of resources, specifically the unwillingness of governments to make adequate provision for community-based facilities, but it is more than this. The de-institutionalisation process affects other groups such as elderly people but it is harder for people with severe mental health problems to find a sense of place and community because the experience of a benign 'inner community' either has never been securely established or, having been established, it has been ruptured and destroyed by subsequent life experience. For many of us the experience of physical isolation and alienation which is so much a part of urban living is made tolerable because, even when alone, we imagine ourselves to be in touch with, in the presence of, a community of others—the family, a group to which we belong, 'my fellow Bengalis', 'my mates down the club' etc. What alternative senses of 'community' exist for those coming out of psychiatric institutions other than 'the community of ex-patients', built upon networks which may well provide an important source of much-needed support?

Improvised communities

Let us now examine a second possible meaning of community mental health. If in reality most neighbourhood communities tend to be either defended or fragmented then we may have to face the fact that the kind of community which policy makers like to talk about—i.e. community as an idealised, warm, benign place to be—is largely mythical. The consolation, however, is this, if good communities cannot be found then at least they can be constructed. Indeed, in my experience, many ex-patients do precisely this. They use existing features of the urban landscape—second-hand shops, flea markets, run down church or community centres—as sites to gather along with many others who may feel themselves to be 'outsiders' in some way or another. Many of these places are 'run' by volunteers, activists or people on employment schemes. Such places provide shelter, a place to be, a space which feels owned by all rather than one belonging to 'them' (i.e. the staff, etc.) and a semblance of purpose which is just sufficient to provide those present with a rationale for being there. For many people such sites do provide a sense of place and hence they constitute one more small community in what is often an already heterogeneous neighbourhood, a community which is accepted if not interacted with by others.

So far I have focused on the way in which ex-patients may often use aspects of the local environment to improvise communities, and clearly many places designed to enable

WHAT IS COMMUNITY MENTAL HEALTH?

individuals to undertake the transition from institutionalised to non-institutionalised life—community houses, day centres, etc.—can also become sites for such real but improvised communities. I have a suspicion, however, that the 'normalisation approach' (embodied in the King's Fund publication *An Ordinary Life*) may lead us to overlook and devalue such possibilities. There is a danger that the desire to return people to a *normal* life within *natural* communities could lead policy makers and mental health workers to consider such group homes and other 'supported' living schemes as somehow unnatural, second best, 'temporary way stations' on the ex-patient's career towards independent living in his/her own flat, etc. As should by now be clear, although such a perspective is undoubtedly well-meaning, I consider it to be mistaken in its assumption that some communities are more genuine and less artificial than others. And in shunning what it may deem to be 'second best' communities, it may condemn individuals to a solitary and isolated life, independence without interdependence. I was reminded of this issue when reading a recent study of the implementation of community mental health policies in London. In this study Tomlinson (1991) reflects on the finding of Perring (1990) that many group homes do indeed resemble 'a sort of alternative community' but one which remains isolated 'within the community' because those running them have not found any way of integrating them into the neighbourhood. I hope that I have established the fact that in many neighbourhood communities 'integration' in the foreseeable future is just not possible, no more possible than the integration of the Bengalis in London's East End. In such situations the effective policy goal should be peaceful cohabitation, or, as Mao might have said, "let a thousand communities grow"!

Finally, the point surely is that service users must always have the right to choose how they wish to live without the professional agenda intruding and, I would add, so long as they are aware of the alternatives if people wish to remain in an environment that others might see as institutionalised then so be it. We need to reflect long and hard on the way in which ideas of asylum, dependency and refuge have become unfashionable and undesirable concepts in today's policy environment.

A healthy community?

The third and last meaning of community mental health I wish to consider is the most difficult and intangible one—what is a (mentally) healthy community and how might the development of such a thing be facilitated? The first point to establish is that although many communities (neighbourhood, ethnic and other communities) may construe themselves to be homogeneous, the reality is that all communities possess a multiplicity of differences. Within the vast majority of communities certain kinds of difference will be experienced as dangerous. Moreover, attempts will be made to control the danger—by isolating it, by suppressing it, by incorporating it, and so on (Cohen, 1985). Of course such fears are based upon phantasy and therefore one way of modifying them is to enable those holding such phantasies to test them against reality. This can be done if the object of fear and the one who is frightened are brought together in an environment which facilitates communication and understanding. I have watched community development workers achieve this when bringing different 'racial' groups together—it requires a certain courage, an ability to handle conflict and a capacity to value people as people in spite of the oppressive behaviour they may engage in and for which the workers may directly confront them. I have also noticed that such fears can be modified where victim and aggressor find themselves in a situation where they are working, playing or struggling together. The fact remains that some communities, for whatever reason, do have a much greater capacity than others to contain differences without becoming paranoid or fragmented. Yet little is known about why this happens in some places and not in others.

PAUL HOGGETT

Only in such communities is the quest for 'integration' realistic rather than mythical. In my experience they are few and far between but well worth struggling for.

Out of sight . . .

I have tried to illustrate that the concept of community is not necessarily one designed to mislead but that there are in fact many forms that community can take. The danger is that policy makers and many practitioners actually only have one of these in mind, a particular species of community which, far from being the norm, is one of the most elusive. One therefore gets the feeling that the powers that be may not know what they are talking about. Indeed although the National Health Service has had many strengths, its ability to respond to and plan for the needs of groups and collectivities has never been one of these. Experimentation with locality management of community health services is still in its infancy and primary care is still built upon the somewhat arbitrary catchment areas of GP practices. The 1990 NHS & Community Care Act threatens to make the effective local co-ordination of community services an even more difficult task, indeed there is a great danger that provision will become increasingly fragmented rendering the idea of a local community of providers a quite unrealisable one. In this context the forms of policy intent sketched at the beginning of this article with their ambitious and comprehensive plans for service users seem incongruous. I hope I have been able to demonstrate that even if the welfare services were in a state to implement such strategies, there are good grounds for believing that they may reflect something more about the values and assumptions of the 'professional classes' than the actual needs of service users and ex-users themselves. Why should users necessarily value 'independence'? And to parody only slightly, why should they prefer the company of 'normal people' to the company of fellow ex-patients or other outsiders? In saying this I am not arguing that no care should be provided at all, rather what I am wary of are forms of intervention which no matter how well intentioned are ultimately intrusive. If you take the phrase 'to look after' in its most literal sense it suggests to me precisely this form of non-intrusive care. My great fear is that much of the current hubris around community mental health and community care actually masks a reality where there is no-one there 'to look after' or keep ex-patients in mind who, as a consequence, may literally disappear without trace.

References

ANDERSON, B. (1983) *Imagined Communities: Reflections on the Origins and Spread of Nationalism* (London, Verso).

BION, W. (1962) *Learning From Experience* (London, Heinemann).

BION, W. (1970) *Attention and Interpretation* (London, Tavistock Publications).

COHEN, S. (1985) *Visions of Social Control* (Cambridge, Polity Press).

GLASS, J. (1989) *Private Terror/Public Life* (New York, Cornell University Press).

HINSHELWOOD, R. (1987) *What Happens in Groups* (London, Free Association Books).

HINSHELWOOD, R. (1989) *Social Possession of Identity*, in: B. RICHARDS (ed.) *Crises of the Self* (London, Free Association Books).

HOGGETT, P. (1989) 'The Labour of Love' and 'a primary social medium': two problematics in contemporary psychoanalysis, *Free Associations*, 15, pp. 87–107.

MURRAY, C. (1984) *Losing Ground: American Social Policy 1950–80*, (New York, Basic Books).

MURRAY, C. (1990) *The Emerging British Underclass* (London, Institute of Economic Affairs).

PERRING, C. (1990) *Leaving the hospital behind? An Anthropological Study of Group Homes in Two London Boroughs* (Unpublished Ph.d. thesis, London School of Economics).

SUTTLES, G. (1972), *The Social Construction of Communities Chicago* (Chicago, University Chicago Press).

TOMLINSON, D. (1991), *Utopia, Community Care and the Retreat From The Asylums* (Milton Keynes, Open University Press).

WILSON, W. (1987) *The Truly Disadvantaged: the Inner City, the Underclass and Public Policy* (Chicago, University of Chicago Press).

VOICES

WINNICOTT, D. W. (1976a) *The Maturational Processes and the Facilitating Environment* (London, Hogarth Press).

WINNICOTT, D. W. (1976b) *The capacity to be alone*, in: D. W. WINNICOTT, *The Maturational Processes and the Facilitating Environment* (London, Hogarth Press).

VOICES

The good team

We were a really good team. It was right at the beginning; we had just started. We'd just had a couple of weeks of an induction course for the new service which had brought us all very close together. We were all very well motivated and of course we were not weighed down by impossible case loads.

The manageress came up and told us that there was an old gent with dementia who had just found his wife dead and was in a terrible state. His wife was not only his wife she had been his major carer and he was well into his dementia. She was the one who had kept the roof over his head, kept him fed, kept him clean, helped him with his confusion. The question for us was how we could keep this old gent in the community and support him through his bereavement without being intrusively and overly managerial. If he'd gone into residential care or respite care it would have been very difficult for him; he'd already lost so many bits and pieces of his memory, bits of his life and now he'd lost his wife; a new domestic and geographical situation would have been completely disorienting and confusing for him.

There were really three teams. There was us the community care workers, then there was the larger team which consisted of the GP, the district nurse, the key worker from the day centre, the key workers from our team and the home help. Then there was the informal neighbourhood team which our community care workers networked into; the relatives were all abroad or far away, but there was a network of friends and neighbours, and then we found his old music friends who later took him out back to some of his old haunts.

Our job as community care workers was to keep the familiar structures as alive and as intact as possible; to make sure that he was physically comfortable and looked after; to help him understand his loss; to be with him as he absorbed it and grieved it; to explain it to him again when he got confused. We also were at the centre of the co-ordination of the efforts of the home help, the district nurse, the GP, the day centre people and the friends. All these needed to be co-ordinated according to the old gent's needs and progress. This involved 24 hour a day care from our community care team for the first week, but by the end of two weeks the old gent's situation had stabilised enormously. We had two key workers for that first intensive week and they were supported by three back-up workers. The larger multiprofessional team met at the beginning and at regular intervals throughout the crisis period to co-ordinate efforts.

It makes you wonder what makes a good team, or series of teams, tick. I think it's a common sense of purpose and a well trained group of professionals who know what their job is, and know what other members of the team can do. The common sense of purpose and the professionalism means everyone understands what they can do and when to do it and when to let someone else from the team do what they can do . . . when to be a support person and when to be the key person. With dementia it's important to have patience and a balanced sense of humour. Having heart is not enough, having a professional approach and understanding is the key. The in-house training that we had had was also important. It shouldn't just happen at the beginning of a new service. You need that kind of education towards a good team dynamic every now and again.

The old gent is dead now. He stayed a further two years in the community and then, as his dementia got worse, he eventually went into a residential home. But he went in in his own time with dignity and not because the bottom had fallen out of his world and residential care was a tidy solution on paper.

Group materials

Questionnaire

The picture of childhood accidents

1 What are the leading causes of death for children of different ages?
Identify the first and second causes of death at each age by writing 1 and 2 in the appropriate boxes.

	under 1 year (excluding 0-4 weeks)	1-4 years	5-14 years
cancer	☐	☐	☐
respiratory diseases	☐	☐	☐
accidents	☐	☐	☐
diseases of the nervous system	☐	☐	☐
congenital anomalies	☐	☐	☐
conditions originating in perinatal period	☐	☐	☐

2 What is the trend in child accident death rates over the past 10-15 years?

☐ increasing
☐ steady
☐ decreasing

3 Which type of accident causes the most fatalities for the ages shown?

● drowning   ● poisoning
● falls   ● transport
● fire and flames   ● suffocation

Write one cause here:

0-1 year   _____
1-4 years   _____
5-9 years   _____
10-14 years   _____

4 What proportion of children attend an Accident and Emergency Department in the course of a year, as the result of an accident? Tick one box.

☐ 1 in 20   ☐ 1 in 6
☐ 1 in 10   ☐ 1 in 3

Group materials

5 What percentage of children attending Accident and Emergency Departments following an accident at home are admitted for treatment?

❏ 1-2%   ❏ 5-10%   ❏ 10-20%

6 What are the three commonest injuries to under fives seen at Accident and Emergency Departments? Tick three boxes for each group.

	0-9 months	9 months - under 5 years
bruises, tenderness, swelling	❏	❏
burns and scalds	❏	❏
concussion	❏	❏
cuts, lacerations, open wounds and grazes	❏	❏
fractures and dislocations	❏	❏
foreign bodies ingested/in orifice	❏	❏
poisoning/suspected poisoning	❏	❏
sprains and strains	❏	❏
no injury diagnosed	❏	❏

7 Road accidents most commonly happen to children (aged 14 and under) when they are:

❏ cycling
❏ pedestrians
❏ passengers in a vehicle
(Tick one box)

8 Where do most fatal accidents take place?

age 0-4:   ❏ at home   ❏ on or caused by transport
age 5-14:   ❏ at home   ❏ on or caused by transport

9 Do girls have more or fewer accidents than boys?

❏ more
❏ about the same
❏ fewer

10 Are children from families in social classes IV and V, more or less likely to die in an accident than those in classes I and II?

❏ more   ❏ about the same   ❏ less

Group materials

Information sheet

1 Leading causes of death for children

In 1988 the leading causes of death in the United Kingdom were:

	1st	2nd	
4 weeks - 1 year	signs, symptoms and ill-defined conditions (46% deaths)	congenital anomalies (16% deaths)	(accidents account for 3% deaths in this age group)
1-4 years	**accidents** (21% deaths)	congenital anomalies (20% deaths)	
5-9 years	**accidents** (34% deaths)	cancer (22% deaths)	
10-14 years	**accidents** (36% deaths)	cancer (17% deaths)	(Sources 1-3)

Variations between Scotland, Northern Ireland and England and Wales are shown on page 32. Until the mid 1940s, infectious diseases were the leading cause of death. Since then, accidents have taken over.

2 Trends in child accident death rates

Answer: Decreasing. Child accident death rates have been decreasing from the late 1940s and particularly for children aged 1-4 years. Hospital statistics show a decline in admissions for children's accidents since 1976 (Source 4). This may reflect changes in admission policies rather than real changes in the incidence of accidents.

3 Types of fatal accident (1988)

Age	0-1	1-4	5-9	10-14
England and Wales	Suffocation (47%)	Transport (34%)	Transport (70%)	Transport (75%)
Scotland	Suffocation (55%)	Fire & flames (41%)	Transport (63%)	Transport (60%)
Northern Ireland	Transport/Falls/ Other (all 33%)	Transport (56%)	Transport (80%)	Transport (59%)
United Kingdom	Suffocation (45%)	Transport (35%)	Transport (70%)	Transport (73%)

(Sources 1-3)

The proportions of different types of accidents at various ages are shown on page 33.

4 Hospital attendance

Answer: England and Wales — 1 in 6. Scotland and Northern Ireland — no data available. Local studies suggest that about one in six children a year attend an Accident and Emergency Department for treatment to accidental injuries (Source 7). Figures for local studies have been used to produce these estimates for England and Wales (Source 5).

Group materials

5 Admissions for treatment

Answer: 5-10% (Source 6).

Most injuries are superficial and need only one visit, some injuries need no treatment at all. The accidents which result in the longest stays in hostpital are road accidents and severe burns and scalds (Source 5). Overall the proportion of the child population (aged 14 and under) admitted for treatment to an accidental injury, in 1988, was:
England and Wales — no data available, Scotland — 1.4% (Source 8), Northern Ireland — 0.6% (Source 9).

6 Commonest injuries to under fives

	0-9 months	9 months - 4 years
1st	bruises, tenderness and swelling (35%)	cuts (47%)
2nd	no injury diagnosed (16%)	bruises (25%)
3rd	cuts, lacerations, open wounds and grazes (15%)	burns and scalds (7%)

These figures are from the Home Accident Surveillance System for 1987 (Source 6). The high proportion of cases where no injury was diagnosed for 0-9 month old children (16%) indicates that when very young children are injured some parents prefer to be cautious and take them to hostpital to be checked over.

7 Road accidents

Answer: Pedestrians.

Road accidents 1988: percentages of children involved in different activities

	England and Wales	Scotland	Northern Ireland
Pedestrians	49%	57%	49%
Car passengers	18%	12%	39%
Pedal cyclists	29%	25%	11%
Other*	4%	6%	0.05%

* includes passengers in a bus, coach, caravan, taxi, motorbike or any other vehicle

(Source 10)

Although road accidents usually account for around 2% of reported accidents to children, they account for 55% of fatalities and 10% of cases requiring hospital admission (Source 5). In 1988 in England and Wales there were just over 37,000 reported road accidents to children aged 14 and under. Of these 1% were fatal, with 19% resulting in serious injury and 80% in slight injury (Source 10). It is widely recognised that there is massive under-reporting to police of accidents to cyclists (Source 5).

Group materials

8 Location of accidents

Answer: Age 0-4 — at home. Age 5-14 — on or caused by transport.

In 1988 in the United Kingdom the percentages of fatalities by location was as follows:

Age	0-4	5-14	total 0-14
Home	55%	16%	31%
Transport related	33%	76%	55%
Other	12%	8%	14%

Figures compiled for the United Kingdom from Sources 2, 3 and 13.

9 Sex differences

Answer: Boys have more accidents than girls at all ages.

The male:female ratio increases with age, for deaths. Emergency admissions to hospital are also more common for boys than for girls.

Number of accidental deaths, by age and sex, 1988

	Age 0-4 boys	girls	Age 5-14 boys	girls
England and Wales	161	123	304	101
Scotland	25	16	47	13
Northern Ireland	2	2	33	19

(Sources 1-3)

10 Socio-economic differences

Answer: More likely.

A review of childhood mortality in the period 1979-80,'82-83, found that children in social classes IV and V had just over twice as many fatal accidents as children in social classes I and II. The biggest differences were for death from fire and flames: five times more children in classes IV and V died in this period, than in classes I and II.

Group materials

Sources

(1) **Mortality statistics, cause, 1988** Series 2, no 15 *OPCS* HMSO London 1990

(2) **Registrar General Scotland, Annual Report 1988** HMSO Edinburgh 1989

(3) **Registrar General Northern Ireland, Annual Report 1988** HMSO Belfast 1989

(4) **Hospital in-patient enquiry** Series MB4, no 27 *DHSS/OPCS* HMSO London 1987

(5) **Basic principles of child accident prevention** *Child Accident Prevention Trust* London 1989

(6) **Home and Leisure Accident Research Eleventh Annual Report Home Accident Surveillance System 1987 Data** *Department of Trade and Industry* London 1989

(7) **Joint statement on children's attendances at Accident and Emergency Departments** *British Paediatric Surgeons and Casualty Surgeon's Association* London 1987 (revised 1988)

(8) Information provided by the Information and Statistics Division, CSA for Scottish Health Service, Edinburgh 1990

(9) Figures prepared for: **Hospital Activity Analysis** *Department of Health and Social Services (Northern Ireland) Statistics Branch*

(10) Analysis provided by the Directorate of Statistics, Department of Transport, London

(11) **Road Traffic Accident Statistics 1988** *Royal Ulster Constabulary* HMSO Belfast 1989

(12) **Deaths by accidents and violence.** Quarterly Monitors DH4 series. *Office of Population Censuses and Surveys* London

(13) **Deaths from accidents and violence** *OPCS* Monitors DH4 88/5/7 and DH4 89/1/2

Child accident death rate, 1988

Note Scotland and Northern Ireland — the actual numbers of accidents, particulary at age 0-1, are small so slight fluctuations in numbers from year to year can result in seemingly large fluctuations to death rates per million of the population. (Sources 1-3)

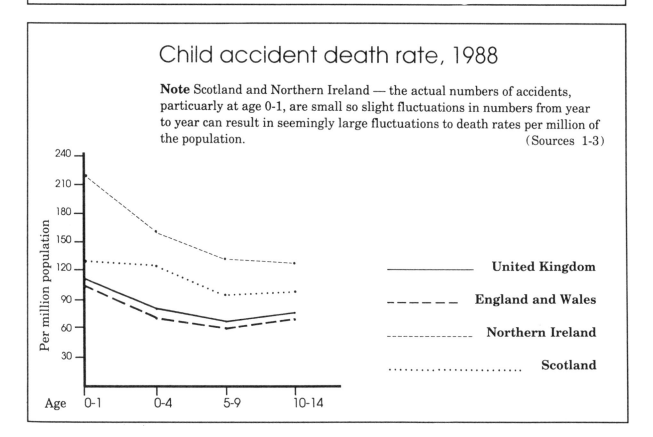

Public Health (1994), **108**, 21–25   © The Society of Public Health, 1994

Children's Safety in the Home: Parents' Possession and Perceptions of the Importance of Safety Equipment

D. Kendrick, MRCGP MFPHM

Lecturer in Public Health Medicine, Department of Public Health Medicine and Epidemiology, University of Nottingham, Medical School, Queen's Medical Centre, Nottingham NG7 2UH

A parental survey was administered by health visitors at the eight-month hearing test in five areas of Nottingham in order to examine possession and perceptions of the importance of safety equipment. The response rate was 82.2%. A sizeable proportion of families were found not to possess items of safety equipment thought to be appropriate for an eight-month-old child. Most items were perceived to be very important with a significant association between perceived importance and possession of equipment ($P = 0.008$). Perceptions of importance did not vary by socio-demographic variables but families on benefit, single-parent families, non-owner-occupiers and families with only one child possessed significantly fewer items. It is concluded that there is considerable scope for educating parents about safety equipment and that the provision of affordable safety equipment schemes should be considered by agencies implementing *The Health of the Nation*.

Introduction

The majority of accidental injuries to children aged under five years occur in the home.[1] In England and Wales 219 children under five died as a result of an accident at home in 1990[2] and it is estimated that there are 645,000 attendances at an accident and emergency department each year following accidental injury.[3] There is evidence that the acquisition and use of safety equipment appropriate to the developmental stage of the child can reduce the incidence of accidental injuries in childhood.[4-7] Parents have identified a need for advice regarding home safety equipment which they consider could be met by the health visitor,[8] and face-to-face contact between health professionals, either doctors[7,9,10] or health visitors[11] has been found to be effective in increasing the acquisition and use of home safety equipment.

As part of the Nottingham Accident Prevention Community Trial, parents have been surveyed to assess their possession and perceived importance of home safety equipment. The resulting information is being used to target home safety advice and to identify families who could benefit from local affordable home safety equipment schemes.

Method

The Nottingham Accident Prevention Community Trial was established in 1990. Health visitors from five geographical areas who had expressed an interest in accident prevention were approached to take part in the trial. The five areas chosen included inner city areas, suburban and rural areas. Three areas received interventions consisting of multi-agency accident prevention training, establishment of local accident prevention groups, local affordable home safety equipment schemes, post-accident

Correspondence to: Dr D. Kendrick. Department of Public Health Medicine and Epidemiology. University of Nottingham. Medical School. Queen's Medical Centre. Nottingham NG7 2UH.

D. Kendrick

follow-up visits by health visitors and community first aid training. The health visitors in the two control areas undertook their usual health visiting which did not include any of the above activities, except for access to an equipment loan scheme, not locally based and poorly funded throughout the period of the project.

The possession and perceptions of importance of home safety equipment were assessed using a specially designed questionnaire, during the period March to April 1992, which was given to all parents attending for their child's eight-month hearing test. This covered socio-demographic variables and possession and perceived importance of fireguards, stairgates, smoke alarms, electric socket covers and car seats: all reported by the Department of Transport, in their booklet *Keep them Safe*[12] to be appropriate to a child with the development of at least eight months of age. Perceptions of importance were recorded on a five-point Likert scale ranging from 'not at all important' to 'very important'. The reliability of the responses has been assessed by a repeat postal questionnaire to a random sample of 20% of the parents attending for the hearing test, posted within two weeks of the attendance. The results have been analysed by socio-demographic variables using χ^2 tests. Where the expected number in a cell was less than 5, Fisher's exact test has been used.

Results

Over the two-month period, 247 parents attended with their children for the hearing test, and 203 parents completed the questionnaire producing a response rate of 82.2%. Eleven questionnaires were unusable due to the parents not entering the child's date of birth. Fifty reliability questionnaires were sent to parents who attended the hearing test and completed a questionnaire; 36 were returned after one mailing. Reliability data are therefore available on 18.8% of the respondents to the original questionnaire. The reliability of the responses was high: 90% of answers concerning possession of safety equipment were concordant with those of the original questionnaire. The reliability of the responses concerning the perceived importance of safety equipment was also high, with 76% of responses concordant with the original response and 94% within one point on the Likert scale of the original response.

The number of families possessing each of the items of safety equipment is shown in Table I. After accounting for individual circumstances some families still possessed few items of equipment, with 12% of families possessing no equipment or only one item.

The reasons cited for not possessing equipment are shown in Table II.

Most families perceived all five items of safety equipment to be very important. Socket covers were least likely to be perceived as very important (63% of parents) whilst stairgates and fireguards were most likely to be perceived as very important (87.5% of parents). There was a significant association ($\chi^2 = 6.95$ with 1 degree of freedom, $P = 0.008$) between perceived importance of and possession of safety equipment. There was no significant difference in perceived importance of safety equipment by any socio-demographic variables (maternal age, number of children, sex of child, housing tenure, receipt of benefits, [other than child benefit], family type or previous accidental injury requiring medical attention). Families in receipt of benefits, non-owner-occupiers, single-parent families and families with only one child were found to possess significantly fewer items of safety equipment (Table III).

Discussion

This study has demonstrated that a significant number of families do not possess items of safety equipment appropriate to the developmental stage of their children. The

D. Kendrick

majority of families perceived all items of safety equipment to be very important for keeping their children safe. As expected there was a strong association between perceived importance and possession of equipment. Families receiving benefits, non-owner-occupiers, single-parent families and families with only one child possessed significantly fewer items of safety equipment than did other families, despite perceiving the possession of safety equipment to be equally important.

There are some methodological issues to deal with before discussing the results further. First, the questionnaire was administered by health visitors at the eight-month hearing test. Consequently responders are a self-selected group of parents in that they have chosen to attend. Non-attenders or parents attending but not completing the questionnaire may possess less safety equipment and perceive it to be of less importance. This would be consistent with the published studies on non-responders to lifestyle surveys which have found a higher prevalence of less 'healthy' behaviour in non-responders.[13,14]

This study demonstrates the scope for educating parents about safety equipment applicable to the developmental stage of their children. Such education has been shown to be effective in terms of acquisition, use of equipment and reduction in the incidence of injuries.[4-7,9,10] Parents recognise the value of such information, along with information on local availability and safety standards.[8] Information about safety equipment should therefore form part of routine child health surveillance programmes undertaken by both health visitors and doctors. Information should also be provided opportunistically on home visits and at acute injury consultations.[15] Health Authorities and Family Health Service Authorities should therefore ensure that child health surveillance programmes incorporate such information.

The finding that possession of equipment varied by socio-demographic variables but perceived importance did not, is concerning. Families at greatest risk of accidental injury[16-18] may be those with most barriers to acquiring equipment such as low income, lack of transport and lack of child care facilities. The provision of locality-based, affordable safety equipment schemes could partly address this issue. As purchasing and installing equipment is not the responsibility of a single agency, obtaining funding for such schemes can be difficult.[19] Second-hand schemes may not be an option because of problems with checking equipment and apportioning responsibility for ensuring equipment is safe. Health Authorities should consider negotiating the funding of such schemes with the various agencies involved in implementing *The Health of the Nation*[20] at a local level. Such debate may test the commitment of agencies to accident prevention and to achieving *The Health of the Nation* targets, but local solutions to such problems will need to be found if the targets are to be reached.

References

1. The Child Accident Prevention Trust (1989). *Basic Principles of Child Accident Prevention.* London: Child Accident Prevention Trust.
2. Office of Population Censuses and Surveys (1990). *Mortality Statistics, Series DH4: Injury and Poisoning, No. 16.* London: HMSO.
3. Department of Trade and Industry (1992). *Home and Leisure Accident Research; 1989 Data, Thirteenth Annual Report of the Home Accident Surveillance System.* London: Department of Trade and Industry.
4. Speigel, C. N. & Lindaman, F. C. (1977). Children can't fly: a programme to prevent childhood morbidity and mortality from window falls. *American Journal of Public Health* **67**, 1143–1147.
5. Reisinger, K. S. (1980). Smoke detectors: reducing deaths and injuries due to fire. *Pediatrics*, **65**, 718–724.

Children's Safety in the Home

Table I Possession of items of safety equipment (percentage)

Equipment	Number (%) of families possessing equipment	Number (%) of families without equipment*
Stairgate	109 (56.8)	75 (39.1)
Fireguard	119 (62.0)	62 (32.3)
Smoke alarm	129 (67.2)	61 (31.8)
Socket covers	119 (62.0)	73 (38.0)
Car seat	137 (71.4)	15 (7.8)

*Excluding families whose circumstances did not require equipment; for example lack of stairs, fires or car or where the parents said that the child was not sufficiently mobile to reach the danger.

Table II Reasons cited for families not possessing safety equipment

Reason cited	No. of times reasons cited
Child unable to reach danger/ not sufficiently mobile	69
No car/fire/stairs	55
Parents not thought about equipment	34
Parents cannot afford equipment	33
Parents planning to get equipment	27
Child always supervised	10
Fire is rarely used	8
Just moved/moving house	8
Other*	37

*Other includes no room in car for car seat (3), socket covers not considered important (3), child aware of danger (3), child not had any accidents yet (2), parents not aware of availability of equipment (2), fireguard not considered necessary for a gas fire (2).

Table III Possession of safety equipment by socio-demographic variables

Socio-demographic variable	Items of safety equipment		Significance
	0–2	3–5	
Receiving benefits	31	39	$\chi^2 = 4.88$ with 1
Not receiving benefits	32	81	degree of freedom. $P = 0.03$
Non-owner-occupier	36	43	$\chi^2 = 12.58$ with 1
Owner-occupier	21	80	degree of freedom. $P = 0.0004$
Single-parent family	16	13	$\chi^2 = 6.06$ with 1
Married/cohabiting	49	107	degree of freedom. $P = 0.01$
Maternal age < 20	3	6	Fisher's exact test. 1-tailed value.
Maternal age ⩾ 20	59	117	$P = 0.65$
Single child	33	40	$\chi^2 = 5.51$ with 1
More than one child	34	85	degree of freedom. $P = 0.02$

Children's Safety in the Home

6. Sorensen, B. (1976). Prevention of burns and scalds in a developed country. *Journal of Trauma*, **16**, 249–258.

7. Guyer, B., Gallagher, S. S., Chang, B. H., Azzara, C. V., Cupples, L. A. & Carlton, T. (1989). Prevention of childhood injuries; evaluation of the state wide childhood injury prevention programme (SCIPP). *American Journal of Public Health*, **79**, 1521–1527.

8. Coombes, G. (1991). *You can't watch them twenty four hours a day; Parents' and Children's Perceptions, Understanding and Experience of Accidents and Accident Prevention*. London: Child Accident Prevention Trust.

9. Miller, R. E., Reisinger, K. S., Blatter, M. M. & Wucher, F. (1982). Pediatric counselling and subsequent use of smoke detectors. *American Journal of Public Health*, **72**, 392–393.

10. Bass, J. L., Mehta, K. A., Ostrovsky, M. & Halperin, S. F. (1985). Educating parents about injury prevention. *Pediatric Clinics of North America*, **32**, 232–242.

11. Colver, A. F., Hutchinson, P. J. & Judson, E. C. (1982). Promoting children's home safety. *British Medical Journal*, **285**, 1177–1180.

12. Child Accident Prevention Trust (1990–91). *Keep them Safe; A Guide to Child Safety Equipment*. London: Child Accident Prevention Trust.

13. Smith, C. & Nutbeam, D. (1990). Assessing non-response bias; a case study from the 1985 Welsh Heart Survey. *Health Education Research*, **5**, 381–386.

14. Bali, B. (1993). A telephone interview follow up of non-responders to a lifestyle survey. B Med Sci dissertation presented to the Department of Public Health Medicine and Epidemiology, Nottingham University Medical School.

15. Sibert, J. R. (1991). Accidents to children; the doctor's role. Education or environmental change? *Archives of Disease in Childhood*, **60**, 890–893.

16. Department of Health and Social Security (1980). *Inequalities in Health: Report of a Research Working Group (The Black Report)*. London: Department of Health and Social Security.

17. Constantinides, P. (1988). Safe at home? Children's accidents and inequality. *Radical Community Medicine*, 31–34.

18. Taylor, B., Wadsworth, J. & Butler, N. R. (1983). Family type and accidents in preschool children. *Journal of Epidemiology & Community Health*, **37**, 100–104.

19. Child Accident Prevention Trust (1991). *Approaches to Local Child Accident Prevention: Home Safety Equipment Loan Schemes*. London: Child Accident Prevention Trust.

20. The Department of Health (1992). *The Health of the Nation*. London: HMSO.

CHILD PROTECTION

Accident prevention: a community approach

Child accidents are the main cause of death and a considerable cause of morbidity in children, as well as anxiety to adults. Attempts to tackle this major health problem have tended to rely on campaigns of education and exhortation; public health strategies remain underdeveloped. Health visitors are well placed to pursue child safety strategies which build on parents' own knowledge and experience. HELEN ROBERTS describes an initiative based not on the question, why did that accident happen? but the more intriguing question of how is it that most parents manage to keep their children safe most of the time and what can we learn from them? *Health visitor 1991; 64, 7: 219-220*

Scotland is in the unenviable position of having one of the worst child accident rates in Europe[1] and within Scotland the data suggest that Glasgow is a particularly dangerous city for a child to inhabit.[2]

The starting point of a great deal of work on child accidents is that children are a danger to themselves and that parents are deficient in their safety-keeping activities. Accidents, according to this approach, happen because children and their parents are not well-enough informed, are not properly competent, or do not have the right safety equipment. A number of urban myths have grown up around the inadequacies of parents as safety keepers and it is suggested that the poor performance of mothers and children can be modified by exhortation and health education. Less attention is given to the poor performance of car drivers, the kitchens planned by people who have clearly never had to supervise a stove and young children at the same time, or architects producing nifty looking balconies with enticing gaps at tiny tot level. Where attention has been drawn to these deficiencies, it has been inadequately used by decision makers.[3,4]

Society is constructed with healthy, resilient, able-bodied adults in mind. The majority of environments are not child-friendly. The puzzle is not 'why do child accidents happen?' but rather, how is it, that under the most unpropitious circumstances, most parents manage to keep their children safe most of the time? And how can we learn from what parents already know about keeping their children safe and build on this? Individual parents, knowing the dangers, respond by avoidance or protection. But their knowledge, when it informs policy, can be used to reduce those external perils. People who live in a particular community are well placed to recognise dangers specific to that community and their own dwellings.

The work described here runs alongside, but is independent from, a parents' action campaign to improve child safety in the community. Corkerhill, where the project is based, is a housing scheme in the south of Glasgow with about 580 dwellings, a predominantly social class IV/V population and high unemployment. Over one quarter of the households with children are headed by a lone parent, and the number of households with four or more children is significantly higher than that for the district or the region as a whole.[5] Social class, large family size, unemployment and single parenthood have been identified as risk factors for child accidents.[6-8] These very factors are also, of course, likely to be associated with hazardous living conditions. This association, though frequently described, has not been adequately explained. In trying to do this, we are working at a local level to:

- identify factors predisposing children to be at risk of, and protected from, accidents in the home and in the wider environment
- investigate the strategies which families adopt to maintain safety and look at the ways in which safety-keeping is incorporated into routine family behaviour.

The research has four components, the first of which has been completed:[9]

- group interviews with parents from different types of dwelling in the area and with teenagers from the community
- work with younger children to establish their view of the precipitants of accidents and near-accidents in their own community
- a household survey to establish the prevalence of child accidents and near accidents in the community studied
- case studies of successful and unsuccessful accident prevention strategies in 20 households.

Group interviews

The starting point for the research was a series of group interviews. Groups of parents were recruited on the basis of the type of housing they lived in and interviewed on three occasions. It was felt that housing type rather than, say, lone parenthood was a more appropriate selection criterion in view of our interest in the role of dwelling design, condition and use in influencing the level of risk or protection which parents have to manage. The group interviews covered what an accident is and who is at risk, the sorts of accidents most common in the community and a description of accidents which nearly happened but were averted. (Safety strategies in aviation and anaesthetics commonly use 'near-misses' to inform policies.) In the second week we explored specific dangers in the home and the community. In the final week we asked the group to put forward their ideas on accident prevention in their own community. By

Helen Roberts DPhil
medical sociologist
Public health research unit (formerly the
Social paediatric and obstetric research
unit),*
University of Glasgow

* The research unit is supported by the Chief scientist office, Scottish home and health department and the Greater Glasgow health board. The opinions expressed in this paper are not necessarily those of the Scottish home and health department.

Professional

asking them to suggest high cost, low cost and no cost strategies, we hope to have a source of data for a positive input to local decision making.

In addition to the three housing-type groups, a teenage group of 13, 14 and 15 year olds was convened and met on three occasions with similar issues addressed. We felt that a teenage perspective would be valuable since this group is young enough to remember accidents and hazards they experienced as children, yet old enough to have taken on child care responsibilities for younger siblings and to have insight into the risk factors which currently exist. A professional perspective on some of the safety problems facing this community was obtained from a group interview with representatives from health visiting, health promotion, housing, environmental health, the police, the roads department and the fire brigade.

Child's eye view

We view this stage of the investigation as experimental and developmental. Work with children in the area of accidents has largely focused on an educational approach. Our perspective is rather different in focusing on children's views of danger and safety *within the particular context of this community*. We also intend to explore children's concepts of accidents; for example, do they see them in terms of 'luck'; how far do they think they are preventable?

The household survey

The household survey will cover all households in Corkerhill with children aged up to and including 14 years. Although data on accidents which lead to death or hospital admission are good, they do not tell us much about the *extent* of the problem. The intention of the survey is to:
- provide population based data on accident prevalence in a specific community
- provide data on factors which frustrate the accident chain by an exploration of near accidents.

The survey will ask, for each child aged 0–14 inclusive, whether there has been an accident over the last 12 months. As a recall device, these will be divided into accidents requiring hospital admission, accidents requiring hospital attention, accidents resulting in a visit to the GP, accidents where attention was not sought from a medical source but there was some injury, accidents where there was no injury, and near-accidents. We are aware of the problem of recall bias here. Parents are more likely to recall an accident resulting in hospital

admission than one they dealt with themselves. Only the more serious accidents requiring no medical attention or near accidents are likely to be recalled. At the design stage and in the pilot study we are giving attention to formulating questions in such a way as to minimise this bias.

On the basis of data obtained from the group interviews, there will also be a series of questions on perceived 'risk factors' in the environment and parents' strategies for maintaining safety.

A number of parents in the community have experience of survey work, having carried out a survey into health problems believed by the community to be related to the use of chemical anti-mould agents in their damp housing. While 'popular epidemiology' studies have been described in the United States[10] we are aware of no such initiatives in the UK. We intend to train ten parents to conduct the 250 interviews on the estate.

'Real accidents'

The case studies are intended to:
- provide detailed examples of the negotiation of safety in practice as one aspect of daily routine
- provide detailed examples of parents' accounts of accidents which have happened, including causes and consequences.

It is clear from the child development literature that risk taking is a normal part of early child development and one of the ways in which the child learns. Given this, an understudied area of child safety is the way in which parents, and mothers in particular, maintain child safety in practice. Twenty illustrative case studies will be carried out, based first on ten extended interviews on safety maintenance. Topics covered will include an exploration of the part played by safety maintenance in family priorities; how safety is managed when there are competing priorities (for example: clothes to be hung out on the washing green and three children in a flat three floors up); how safety is managed when there is a break in routine or interruptions to routine. The second set of ten case studies will be based on accidents which have actually happened and which have been identified either through the group interviews or the survey. These will describe in some detail the circumstances of an accident; the child's view of why it happened; the views of the parents and subsequent preventive action taken, if any.

Each of the four components of the research is expected to make a contribution to our understanding of child accidents and together these differing methodologies present a way of exploring safety as a social value in a particular community.

Discussion

The Corkerhill parents' campaign on child accidents is community led and they are partners in the research in more than a superficial sense. They have been involved in the planning and organisation; theoretically the research is founded in the experiences of the community; materially, both interviewers and group respondents are being compensated for their time.

A number of expert groups have been drawn into this project including the local police, the health promotion department of the health board, workers with young people and drugs and the local health council. The parents' group is actively trying to forge links with the district and regional councils, from whom they hope to obtain some modest funds and, equally importantly, make the politician and officer links which will enable the successful elements of this project to be used and adapted elsewhere in the city. While the community is aware that neither we nor they will be able to provide a knitting pattern for safety, we expect to provide a basis for safety at home, at play and in transit at the community level. The combination of the research project and the parents' action is one we feel may be an effective way of producing local safety data, exploring practical ways of putting our findings into practice and disseminating them to other communities ■

References

1 Blondel B *et al.* Mortalité des enfants de 1 à 4 ans dans les pays de la communauté europééne. *Archive françaises de pédiatrie* 1985; 42: 645–9.
2 Strathclyde Regional Council. Child pedestrian casualties in areas of priority treatment. Glasgow: SRC, 1987.
3 Sinnott R, Jackson H. Developments in house and home safety. Coventry: University of Warwick, 1990.
4 Ranson R. Home safety — the challenge to public health. Coventry: University of Warwick, 1987.
5 Strathclyde Regional Council. Voluntary population survey, 1987.
6 Wadsworth J *et al.* Family type and accidents in pre-school children. *Journal of Epidemiology and Community Health* 1987; 37: 100–4.
7 Sibert J. Stress in families of children who have ingested poisons. *British Medical Journal* 1975; 3,5975: 87–9.
8 Brown G and Davidson S. Social class, psychiatric disorder of mother and accidents to children. *Lancet*, 1978, 1,8060: 378–80.
9 Roberts H, Smith S, Lloyd M. Safety as a social value. Glasgow: Public health research unit, 1991.
10 Brown G. Popular epidemiology: community response to toxic waste induced disease. In: Konrad P, Kern R. The sociology of health and illness: critical perspectives. New York: St Martin's Press, 1990.

The project was carried out jointly with Susan Smith, professor of human geography, University of Edinburgh and the group interviews were funded by The Nuffield Foundation.

THE
HEALTH
OF THE NATION

July 1993

PURCHASING FOR *THE HEALTH OF THE NATION*

One year on from the launch of *The Health of the Nation* strategy there is encouraging evidence from all regions of its influence on service contracts with local providers. Publications such as the Key Area Handbooks and *First Steps in the NHS* gave recommendations of good practice and effective interventions which have been incorporated into many service specifications. There are also many examples of resource shifts and of new and flexible clinic services, particularly for young people.

Here we show examples from 1993/4 purchasing contracts throughout the country of the wide range of innovations and initiatives to pursue the health strategy.

These examples show health objectives becoming firmly embedded in the management processes of the new NHS. This momentum will be sustained into 1994/5 with *The Health of the Nation* identified as one of the top priorities for the NHS in the annual Priorities and Planning Guidance, published at the end of June as EL(93) 54.

The guidance requires regional health authorities to agree with the NHS management executive targets for health improvement, and also milestones towards achieving those targets for stocktaking progress against the strategy in 1995, 1998 and 2001.

Local targets for health improvement are to be agreed between regional health authorities, district health authorities and family health services authorities. Taken together, these local targets should achieve the regional targets and milestones. Although all those working in primary care are essential to the success of the initiative, NHS authorities are asked to specify the particular role of GP fundholders.

The guidance also requires NHS authorities to work on building effective alliances for health and improve the health of their own staff with the development of the Health at Work in the NHS initiative.

NORTHERN

North Durham HA has supplemented its health promotion contract by £25,000 for the development of activities to reduce smoking in young women. There is a £20,000 reserve to fund dietetic services and a £60,000 reserve to improve access to radiotherapy services. The purchasing strategy for elderly people will be revised, stressing the need to focus on accident prevention.

In the 1993/4 contract for **South Durham HA**, a new health promotion campaign has been launched on sexual health. There are also plans to improve the dermatology service for skin cancers and for a multi-disciplinary audit of all suicides and undetermined deaths of people with mental health problems to take place shortly.

Developmental work in **Northumberland HA** includes a health shop on mental health; work in schools to reduce teenage pregnancies and funding for an interagency child accident prevention group.

There are contract agreements to develop locally accessible mental health services in Tyneside and also to make tangible progress on the Health at Work in the NHS initiative. Separate regional strategies are looking at services for mentally disordered offenders.

YORKSHIRE

West Yorkshire HA has increased expenditure on cardio-thoracic surgery at Killingbeck Hospital and Leeds General Infirmary. At **Scunthorpe Community Trust,** an additional psychiatrist has been appointed to focus on deliberate self-harm and suicide.

North Yorkshire HA has an agreement with providers for cardiology services to reflect the monitoring issues around *The Health of the Nation* and £75,000 has been invested by **Bradford HA** for health promotion in 1993/4 through the Bradford "Heartsmart Project".

An accident and prevention co-ordinator has been appointed by **Wakefield HA** to work with local trusts and the community.

Leeds Healthcare has set up a needle exchange scheme through the FHSA and a research project on take-up of cervical smears. A cardiac liaison nurse has been appointed by **East Riding HA** to work between primary and secondary care.

TRENT

Barnsley HA has invested resources in a heart attack response audit aiming to reduce time delays at the district general hospital and has appointed a cardiac arrest resuscitation training officer. A senior dietician will target schools and workplaces and there are plans for a special symptomatic breast screening clinic. In addition, the mental illness day hospital hopes to extend its opening from 5 to 7 days a week.

North Derbyshire HA employs a liaison nurse to work with discharged CHD patients and also aims to reduce teenage smoking through school nursing in Chesterfield. Child safety equipment is being provided to low income families in Bolsover and £10,000 has been made available for healthy workplace initiatives in local firms. Contracts for local providers have included no-smoking and alcohol policy clauses since April 1993.

There is evidence of action on the *First Steps* recommendations in each key area in **Sheffield HA's** service agreements for 1993/4. For example, A & E services will provide health promotion material in minority languages on accident prevention. The contract with the Community and Priority Services Unit specifies implementation of a family planning review and the service agreement for breast screening with Sheffield University Hospital Trusts contains targets specifying levels of uptake and detection rates for cancer.

Leicestershire HA's contracts have a range of *Health of the Nation* measures, including additional investment in mental illness and the enhancement of genito-urinary medicine.

EAST ANGLIA

Supporting local GPs, an additional community dietician has been appointed in **Huntingdon HA.** More funds have been invested in paramedic training for ambulance crews and there is support for local employers in their implementation of no-smoking policies. Child and psychiatry services have received additional resources for improvements, and **Suffolk HA** has increased the number of coronary artery bypass grafts.

Cambridge HA requires all providers to have no-smoking policies in place. There are a growing number of clinics to promote sexual health for young people with Saturday morning sessions taking place in Cambridge each week.

NORTH WEST THAMES

North West Hertfordshire has a contract with the health promotion unit and the general hospitals unit to provide a smoking in pregnancy reduction programme and there is a new genito-urinary clinic with extended opening hours. The health promotion unit has expanded to cover accident prevention.

Similarly, in **South West Hertfordshire** an intensive stop smoking programme has been introduced for pregnant women and there are Look After Your Heart courses for ethnic minority communities.

Barnet HA is buying more episodes of care from Harefield Hospital Trust (the main provider of heart disease treatment in the area) and radiotherapy and chemotherapy from Mount Vernon Hospital Trust (the main provider of cancer services).

Ealing, Hammersmith and Harrow mental health providers are taking part in a multi-disciplinary audit of suicides and there are open access dermatology outpatients sessions with GPs as part of the "Spot the Spot" campaign.

NORTH EAST THAMES

New River HA has allocated £10,000 to implement the Monk Report and *Health of the Nation* recommendations for genito-urinary medicine services and a Saturday morning drop-in centre offering advice on sexual health to young people, has been set up in Colchester by **North Essex HA**.

Redbridge and Waltham Forest has appointed a health promotion officer to co-ordinate healthy lifestyle projects in local schools.

SOUTH EAST THAMES

A no-smoking programme and an alcohol strategy has been introduced by **East Sussex HA** as well as skin cancer prevention programmes; home loan schemes for safety equipment; a suicide prevention programme and a multi-agency HIV/AIDS strategy.

Bexleyheath HA has set targets to improve the uptake of breast screening in primary care. It has also developed protocols with GPs and local mental health services for the treatment of mental health problems, and, as part of the multi-agency strategy for reducing CHD, protocols have also been developed for rehabilitation.

Contracts for providers in **Solihull and Birmingham** now include Health at Work objectives and codes of practice for smoking, food, alcohol and HIV.

MERSEY

A smoking cessation programme has been offered to all NHS employees and staff in primary care in **Liverpool HA.**

In **Wirral HA,** an eleven point strategy for reducing CHD involves the allocation of £50,000 to extend rehabilitation services which has also attracted £350,000 capital from urban aid money. The Stroke Association has been contracted to provide advice, health promotion and therapies for stroke victims and the staff on the rehabilitation team have been increased. £250,000 has been invested to develop projects in primary and community care such as smoking cessation campaigns.

NORTH WESTERN

£75,000 has been allocated to *Health of the Nation* initiatives in **Blackpool, Wyre and Fylde HA** for projects such as a mobile breast screening unit in Preston and a pilot project for contraceptive and safe sex advice for young people.

In **Bury and Rochdale HA**, each provider must have clear healthy employer objectives on smoking, healthy eating, alcohol and exercise.

Oldham HA has appointed a skin cancer co-ordinator and agreed an accident action plan with other voluntary and statutory agencies, focusing on, for example, water safety, playground accidents and fires. The authority also requires patient medical records to include smoking, alcohol and blood pressure information.

Manchester Districts have drawn up an action plan of eleven objectives, covering all key areas, which will be incorporated into the overall purchasing strategy.

These are just some of the initiatives and examples from across the country showing how *The Health of the Nation* strategy is influencing local purchasing strategies. There are of course many others, and there will be more as the strategy is developed in 1994/5.